MRI Physics for Radiologists

Alfred L. Horowitz

MRI Physics for Radiologists

A Visual Approach

Third Edition

With 117 Illustrations

Springer-Verlag
New York Berlin Heidelberg London Paris
Tokyo Hong Kong Barcelona Budapest

Alfred L. Horowitz, M.D.
Magnetic Resonance Imaging
Resurrection Hospital, Chicago, IL
and
Clinical Assistant Professor of Radiology
University of Illinois Hospital at Chicago, Chicago, IL
USA

Library of Congress Cataloging-in-Publication Data
Horowitz, Alfred L.
    MRI physics for radiologists : a visual approach / Alfred L.
Horowitz — 3rd ed.
        p.   cm.
    Includes bibliographical references and index.
    ISBN 0-387-94372-2. — ISBN 3-540-94372-2
    1. Magnetic resonance imaging. 2. Medical physics. I. Title.
    [DNLM: 1. Magnetic Resonance Imaging. 2. Health Physics. WN
    4456 71816m]
    RC78.7.N83H45   1994   94-33017
    538'.36—dc20

Printed on acid-free paper.

Production managed by Laura Carlson; manufacturing supervised by Jacqui Ashri.
Camera-ready copy prepared from the author's Microsoft® Word files.
Printed and bound by R.R. Donnelley & Sons, Harrisonburg, VA.
Printed in the United States of America.

9 8 7 6 5 4 3 2 1

ISBN 0-387-94372-2 Springer-Verlag New York Berlin Heidelberg
ISBN 3-540-94372-2 Springer-Verlag Berlin Heidelberg New York

To my family

Preface

Having struggled with the concepts of magnetic resonance imaging over the years that span the three editions of this book, I find myself arriving at the following conclusion: although the book is ostensibly about physics, it is also a kind of mathematics book. This is not to say that I have suddenly added all sorts of MRI mathematics to this version. Nothing of the kind. What I mean is that in order to understand the principles of MR imaging, one must successfully navigate through an elaborate structure whose essence is very much like a mathematical subject. I say this because as I think about the various topics that are covered in the book, I realize that it is not so much the factual information regarding these topics that is so important, but rather how they relate to each other. The basis for this structure consists of the fundamentals covered in Sections I and II. The miscellaneous subjects of Section III can almost be derived from the first two sections, much as a corollary follows from a theorem.

I wish to emphasize that although the explanations in this book rely heavily on graphics, the text is equally important. I have labored over each paragraph in terms of choice of words and sequence of ideas in order to maximize the clarity of the topics presented. In short, this is meant to be a *teaching* book.

This edition differs from the previous in several respects. First of all, the section on magnetic resonance angiography has been expanded to become a separate chapter and now includes an extensive discussion of phase contrast angiography. Second, an entire chapter has been added covering the nature of matrix size, field of view, and how they influence the quality of the image. There is now a concise explanation of fast spin-echo (or echo planar) imaging as well as greater coverage of the concept of k-space.

I wish to thank Robert Kriz, M.S., Physicist, Department of Radiology, University of Illinois Hospital, for his help on the chapter on matrix size and image quality, as well as all those who have helped to make the first two editions possible.

So once again I will state the purpose and philosophy of this book: to provide a teaching text—an organized, carefully thought out exposition of the principles of MRI and how they interrelate without the use of sophisticated engineering mathematics.

Contents

Section II. The Image in Space

Section III. Miscellaneous Topics

SECTION I
Image Contrast

1
Overview

This book is divided into three major sections. The first two sections treat the fundamental principles of magnetic resonance imaging (MRI): (1) the study of how we obtain tissue contrast, i.e., what makes one tissue appear brighter than another; and (2) the study of how the signals produce an image in space, i.e., what the pattern of these different intensities is. These first two divisions are based on the spin-echo acquisition, which is still the work-horse technique for most MR centers. The third section deals with a number of important miscellaneous topics, which include a study of other techniques, such as fast scans, as well as a consideration of motion and MR angiography (MRA). It is the author's contention that if the reader thoroughly grasps the first two sections, the topics in section three will fall neatly into place. So let us begin with the first area: how we create tissue contrast in MRI.

MRR

"MRI" stands for "magnetic resonance imaging". If we simply change one letter, we obtain a new abbreviation that allows us to easily conceptualize the sequence of events that occurs during magnetic resonance. By substituting "R" for "I", we get "MRR", which stands for:

- MAGNETIC FIELD
- RADIO-FREQUENCY PULSE
- RELAXATION

These three items, taken in that order, represent the chronological sequence of events that occurs whenever a patient undergoes a magnetic resonance imaging procedure: (1) first the patient is placed in a magnetic field; (2) then a radio frequency pulse is applied; and (3) then the pulse is terminated, allowing relaxation to occur.

If we can thoroughly understand each of these topics, then we can comprehend how the magnetic resonance signals are generated and how we are able to obtain images showing tissue contrast. So let us now consider each item in detail.

Before proceeding to the topic of the magnetic field, which is a vector entity, we should next discuss the concept of the vector.

Vectors

A **vector** is a mathematical entity which has magnitude and direction. A **scalar** is a mathematical entity which has only magnitude.

In order for a mathematical element to have direction, it must be multidimensional, and in order for an element to be multidimensional, it must have more than one coordinate. This is why a two dimensional vector might be written as (2,3) and a three dimensional vector would be (4,6,-8), etc.; whereas a scalar is just a quantity, and would simply be written as a number, like "12". (Actually, we could think of scalars as one dimensional vectors.)

For the principles of MRI, we only need two and three dimensional vectors. In order to understand how to represent them pictorially, we will consider two dimensional vectors. Very simply, we graph two dimensional vectors on a Cartesian coordinate system by placing an arrow with its tail at the origin (intersection of the x-y axis) and its head at the coordinates that represent the vector. The magnitude of the vector is the length of the arrow regardless of its direction. Referring to fig. 1.1, the vectors (1,2) and (2,1) are graphed. Note that their magnitudes are the same, although they point in different directions.

Examples of vectors in physics include forces, fields, velocity and acceleration. Distance, volume, and energy are all scalar quantities.

For the remainder of this book, we will distinguish between "axis" and "direction" as illustrated in fig. 1.2 below.

Vector a and vector b are in the same axis, but point in opposite directions. Some use the term "sense" to mean "direction" as we have defined it.

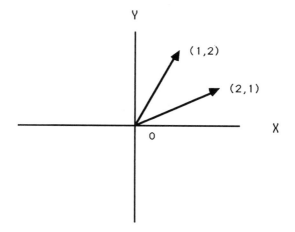

FIG. 1.1- GRAPH OF 2 DIFFERENT VECTORS OF EQUAL MAGNITUDE

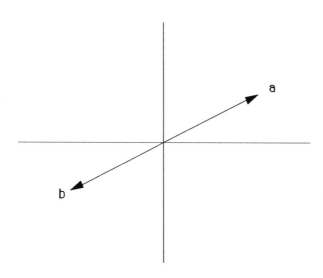

FIG. 1.2- DIRECTION vs. AXIS

2
Magnetic Field

Before we consider magnetic fields, let us first define what a field is in general.

Fields

A **field** is a region in space such that if certain objects are placed within this region, they will experience a force. A field can be considered as a sort of potential force.

The term "certain objects" refers to anything that produces the same sort of field. Hence forces result when two or more similar fields interact.

In classical Newtonian physics, there are three basic forces that are encountered: gravitational, electrical, and magnetic. Each of these forces is associated with a field.

A **magnetic field** is induced if and only if there is a moving electrical charge.

Now we should understand that technically, the direction and axis of the magnetic field vector is **not** the same as that for the magnetic force exerted on an object. In fact, the direction of the magnetic field is perpendicular to both the direction of the magnetic force and the velocity of the moving electrical charge involved in creating the magnetic field. Exactly how this is determined is well explained in most standard high school physics textbooks, but we will not cover it here, because it is not necessary for what we need to know about MRI physics. For the remainder of this text, we will be referring only to the axis and direction of the magnetic field itself.

Basic Types of Magnets

We encounter two types of magnets in every day life: electromagnets and permanent magnets. Electromagnets result when a current is sent through a wire; and permanent magnets are composed of atoms and molecules, which behave like tiny magnets that are all aligned in one direction to produce a net measurable resultant magnetization. The reason each atom or molecule is like a magnet is that each is composed of moving electrical charges: positively charged spinning nuclei and negatively charged spinning electrons. Hence we can see that both electromagnets and permanent magnets produce a magnetic field in accordance with the requirement that every magnetic field be caused by moving electrical charges.

Corresponding to the two types of magnets discussed above, there are two basic types of magnets used in today's MRI scanners: permanent and super-conducting.[*]

Permanent Magnet

A permanent type of MRI scanner utilizes a horseshoe magnet with its poles bent around to face each other (fig. 2.1a). The patient then lies between the poles of the magnet, and the magnetic field travels through the patient from front to back (like an antero-posterior radiograph).

This type of magnet is, of course, always "on".

We measure the strength of a magnetic field in terms of either **Tesla** or **Gauss**. These are units of "magnetic induction". The Tesla is the unit associated with the mks (meters-kilograms-seconds) metric system and the Gauss is associated with the cgs (centimeters-grams-seconds) metric system. One Tesla (abbreviated 1T) equals 10000 Gauss.

The strength of the magnetic field of a permanent type MRI magnet is usually less than .4T.

Super-Conducting Magnet

We said that a moving charge produces a magnetic field. Therefore, if we run an electric current through a wire, we produce a magnetic field. If the wire is wound in a tight helical coil, then we induce a magnetic field whose direction is parallel to the long axis of the coil. This is what is done by those manufacturers

---

[*] There are also "resistive" magnets, which are simply electromagnets that are not superconducting.

who make a super-conducting MRI magnet. The patient lies inside the coil, and the magnetic field runs parallel to the long axis of the patient (fig. 2.1b).

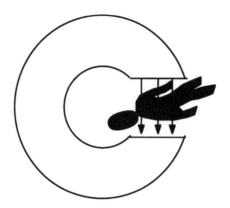

Fig. 2.1a- PERMANENT MAGNET
The arrows indicate the direction of the magnetic field.

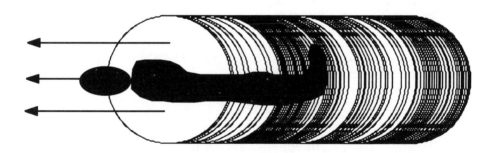

Fig. 2.1b- SUPER-CONDUCTING MAGNET
The arrows indicate the direction of the magnetic field.

Since this magnetic field is produced by an electric current, there is also an **electrical** field. Hence there are two fields produced simultaneously: (1) an electrical field due to the fact that charged particles (electrons) are simply present; and (2) a magnetic field due to the fact that charged particles are **in motion.** We call this an "electromagnetic field". If we place either a charged particle or a magnetic substance in an electromagnetic field, it will experience a force.

Now, in order to create strong electromagnetic fields, we must use large currents. However, because of resistance in the wire, any current will produce heat, and therefore, large currents will result in dissipation of the magnetic field through heat loss.   Therefore, it is necessary to make the entire system extremely cold, and this is done using the "cryogens" liquid helium and liquid nitrogen. Liquid helium is much colder than liquid nitrogen and is used to bring the temperature of the system down to near absolute zero (0° Kelvin or -270 C°). At these low temperatures, there is virtually no resistance in the wires, and hence strong currents can be applied without producing much heat. This process is known as "super-cooling" and electromagnets that are super-cooled are termed "super-conducting magnets".

Liquid nitrogen, which is not nearly as cold as liquid helium, is used to insulate the liquid helium coils to prevent them from equilibrate their temperatures with the environment and thus "boiling off".

Commercial super-conducting magnets range in strength from .35T to 2.0T with most of the modern scanners utilizing a .5 to 1.5T magnet. Hence we can obtain much stronger magnetic fields with a super-conducting magnet than we can with a permanent magnet.

In addition to the fact that super-conducting magnets can be made to be considerably more powerful than permanent magnets, a fundamental difference exists in their operation in that the directions of the fields for the two types of magnets are perpendicular to each other: the permanent magnetic field runs through the patient in an antero-posterior direction, whereas the super-conducting magnetic field runs longitudinally through the patient from head to foot.

Since the vast majority of commercially available MRI scanners make use of super-conducting magnets, we will use the magnet as our prototype for the remainder of this text.

Paramagnetic, Diamagnetic, Ferromagnetic

Let us now consider the effect the magnetic field has on the patient. It is interesting to note that **all** substances are influenced to a greater or lesser extent by a magnetic field. We can classify substances according to the type of effect that the field has on them. If we consider the fact that magnetic fields vary in intensity from one point to another, then we can obtain the following definitions: **paramagnetic** substances are weakly attracted towards the stronger region of a magnetic field. These substances have an unpaired electron in their valence orbits. **Diamagnetic** substances are weakly repelled away from the stronger region of the magnetic field. Diamagnetic substances are essentially non-magnetic substances. The paramagnetic and diamagnetic categories include only atoms and molecules. **Ferromagnetic** substances are **strongly** attracted towards the stronger region of the magnetic field. It is ferromagnetic substances that can remain "magnetized" after the magnetic field is withdrawn. There are essentially only three ferromagnetic elements in nature: iron (Fe), nickel (Ni) and cobalt

(Co). The ferromagnetic category applies to macromolecular crystalline substances.*

Angular Momentum–Nuclear Spin

Of the many paramagnetic substances in the body, it is the hydrogen nucleus that is the substance of most interest to us. This is the substance that is "imaged" in nearly all MRI procedures at this point in time. Nuclear magnetic resonance can occur with any number of nuclei, including ^{1}H, ^{14}N, ^{31}P, ^{13}C, and ^{23}Na. These nuclei all have a "nuclear spin"–that is, they can be thought of as spinning around their axes the way the earth turns around its axis. Elements which have a nuclear spin have an odd number of protons, neutrons, or protons plus neutrons. In more technical physical language, this nuclear spin is referred to as "angular momentum". Only nuclei with angular momentum are candidates for nuclear magnetic resonance. We use the hydrogen nucleus because it is the most abundant and because it yields the strongest MR signal. Hence, although nearly all substances are either paramagnetic, diamagnetic or ferromagnetic, it is only those elements with a nuclear spin that are capable of experiencing nuclear magnetic resonance.

Note that it is misleading to equate the term "proton imaging" with "hydrogen nucleus imaging", for when we do hydrogen nucleus MRI, we are not utilizing protons in other elements.

Magnetic Dipole Moment

Since we are only concerned with NMR (nuclear magnetic resonance) of hydrogen nuclei, we will confine our attention only to that substance from now on. Since the hydrogen nucleus is a spinning charged particle (the positive charge of one proton) we have the situation in which there is a moving charge. Now remember that moving charges produce magnetic fields. Therefore, each hydrogen nucleus is associated with its own minute magnetic field, which is technically termed a "magnetic dipole moment" (MDM). Note the nice relationship between angular momentum and magnetic dipole moments:

> When a nucleus spins, it has **angular momentum**; and when that spinning nucleus has a net charge, then it also has a **magnetic dipole moment.**

---

* There are three other less commonly encountered categories: ferrimagnetism, antiferromagnetism and superparamagnetism. This is very nicely covered by Saini, et. al. in the April, 1988 *AJR.*, and will not be covered here.

We can therefore picture the MDM of each hydrogen nucleus as a tiny bar magnet; and in the presence of the strong magnetic field of a MRI magnet, these minute bar magnets tend to align themselves in the direction of the main magnetic field.   Actually, only one or two per million of these MDM's align themselves with the field; yet that is enough to yield a magnetic resonance signal, as we will see.

Fig. 2.2 illustrates this process by showing the random direction of the MDM vectors when no magnetic field is present as well as their vertical alignment in the presence of the field. Note, of course, that we are over-simplifying in as much as we show **all** the vectors vertically aligned instead of just one or two per million!

Resultant M Vector

Now, since all the vertically aligned MDM vectors point in the same direction, the mathematical laws governing vector addition allow us to combine all those vectors into one long vector representing the linear sum of all those little ones. This gives us a single resultant vector which we can think of as representing the patient's magnetization. (Actually, it is the magnetization of the magnetic dipole moments of the hydrogen nuclei in the patient.) We will call this resultant hydrogen MDM vector the "M" vector. In the next chapter, we will see how the radiofrequency pulse alters this resultant vector.

It is very important for the reader to realize that in this discussion of the alignment of magnetic dipole moments, we have rendered a simplification (not **over**-simplification!) of the physics. A more sophisticated treatment of this subject would involve quantum mechanics (and many readers may have already read such approaches) which consider the MDM's as either parallel (pointing up) or anti-parallel (pointing down). It is the author's firm belief that the more classical approach taken in this book will yield an understanding of the physics of MRI which is entirely adequate for our point of view. Furthermore, since no one can actually *watch* what the nuclei are doing, we develop **constructs** which give us a framework for establishing an understanding of the observed physical phenomena. Both the classical and quantum mechanics approaches are examples of such constructs. We are simply choosing that construct which is appropriate for our purpose, and it will not hinder our understanding of the physical principles as we proceed.

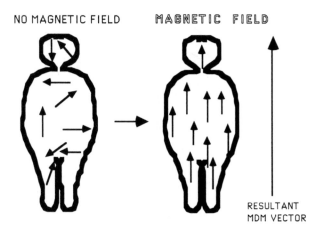

NO MAGNETIC FIELD   MAGNETIC FIELD

RESULTANT
MDM VECTOR

FIG. 2.2- MDM VECTORS INSIDE AND OUTSIDE THE MAGNETIC FIELD

Precession and the Larmor Equation

Now, we have completed our discussion of the magnetic field with the exception of one apparently small embellishment. However, this "embellishment" constitutes one of the most important principles of MRI. Each magnetic dipole moment is "precessing". This means that the "tail" of each vector is stationary, whereas the head is revolving (fig. 2.3). This results in a kind of wobbling motion. This same wobbling motion, or precession, is seen when we spin a top. The top spins around its axis, while the "plane" of the spinning top precesses (somewhat more slowly) around the same axis. The precession of a top is due to the fact that the force of gravity acts perpendicular to the plane of the spinning top. Note the very similar analogy to the NMR case: the hydrogen nucleus is spinning, the MDM is precessing, and the external magnetic field is acting perpendicular to the plane of the spinning nucleus. In a sense, it is gravity that causes the top to process, and the external magnetic field which causes the MDM to precess. However, the analogy is not complete, for in the case of the top, the top is doing both the spinning **and** the precessing; whereas in the NMR case, the hydrogen nucleus is spinning, but it is the MDM which is doing the precessing. However, the analogy is useful to help us picture what is happening at the nuclear level.

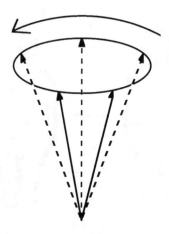

FIG. 2.3- PRECESSING MAGNETIC DIPOLE MOMENT (MDM)

Now here comes the important part:

> The precession frequency (f) of the magnetic dipole moment of a spinning
> nucleus in a magnetic field is given by the equation: $f = \gamma M$, where f is the
> frequency in revolutions per second, M is the strength of the magnetic field in
> Tesla, and γ is the gyro magnetic ratio or constant for the nucleus in question.
> This is the **"Larmor Equation".**

The Larmor equation tells us that the precession rate of the MDM's for a given
nucleus is directly proportional to the strength of the magnetic field. This, of
course, means that if we double the magnetic field strength, then we will also
double the frequency of the precessing MDM's. In a 1.5T MRI scanner,
hydrogen nuclei MDM's are precessing at about 64 MHz (64,000,000
revolutions or cycles per second—note that the term "Hz" means cycles per
second). According to the Larmor equation, these same MDM's would precess
at about 21 MHz if they were in a .5T MRI scanner.

It is important to realize that although hydrogen MDM's precess at 64 MHz in a
1.5T scanner, **other** species of MDM's will precess at totally different rates at
that same magnetic field strength. This will be determined by the gyro magnetic
ratio for each nucleus. Hence, although the gyro magnetic ratio (γ) is constant
for a given nucleus, it varies from nucleus to nucleus. The implication of this is
that when the patient is placed in the scanner, every nuclear species with angular
momentum has MDM's which are precessing at different rates-**all
simultaneously**. Therefore, we must imagine the patient containing many
different varieties of "tops"—all precessing at different rates dictated by their
nuclear species. The hydrogen MDM's constitute only one kind out of many. In

the next chapter, we will see how we **select** the hydrogen MDM's using the radio-frequency pulse.

The reason the Larmor equation is so important is that it describes a very simple **dependence** of the MDM precession frequency on the strength of the magnetic field. Later, we will see that by altering the precession frequencies of the MDM's, we can differentiate between tissue signals as well as spatially encode their locations, which is, of course, the essence of the imaging process. **Since the precession frequencies depend on the magnetic field, the goal of imaging can be accomplished by simply manipulating the external magnetic field.**

Now, we have completed the section on the magnetic field–the "M" of "MRR". In summary, when the patient is placed in the magnetic field, the MDM's of those nuclei with angular momentum align with the direction of the magnetic field and precess with a frequency directly proportional to the strength of the field.

3
Radiofrequency Pulse

We are now ready to begin part two of "MRR"–the radiofrequency pulse (or "RF pulse"). Remember from the first chapter that when we send an electric current through a wire, we create an electromagnetic field. That is, we have both an electrical field and a magnetic field at the same time, which means that either a charged particle or a "magnetizable" substance would experience a force when placed in this region. Now if we make that current an *alternating* current, then at any spatial point in the field, the strength of the field will be varying in time. This means that the force that either a charged particle or a magnetizable substance would experience will vary in time from a maximum in one direction to a maximum in the opposite direction. It turns out that this variation in time can be mathematically described with a simple sine or cosine function.

Electromagnetic Waves

Now it is also the case that this electromagnetic field is propagated through space, i.e., it spreads three dimensionally from one spatial point to another. This takes place at the speed of light. When an electromagnetic field is propagated in this manner, it is termed a "**wave**." To picture this process, just think of what happens when a stone is dropped in a pond. We would see enlarging concentric circles, which represent, in this case, waves in two dimensions (fig. 3.1a). Simply extend this scenario one more dimension to represent enlarging concentric **spheres** in space, and we then have the propagation of an electromagnetic wave (fig. 3.1b).

To summarize what we have just said, when we send an alternating current through a wire, we produce an **electromagnetic field** which propagates through space as an **electromagnetic wave**. These wave characteristics would not exist if the current were not alternating. Note that the electromagnetic field produced by the magnet is a **direct** current, and hence this magnetic field does not vary as a function of time, and there is no electromagnetic *wave* associated with it.

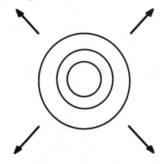

FIG. 3.1a- WAVES IN A POND: EXPANDING CONCENTRIC CIRCLES

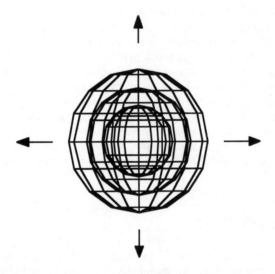

FIG. 3.1b- RF WAVES IN SPACE: EXPANDING CONCENTRIC SPHERES

Periodic Functions

A wave is a cyclic phenomenon, and every wave has a period, a frequency, and an amplitude. The "period" of a wave is the time it takes for the wave to complete one full cycle, and it has the units of time (seconds, minutes, etc.); the "frequency" of a wave is the reciprocal of the period (1/period), and it has the units of 1/time (sec^{-1} or min^{-1}), usually referred to as "cycles per second", etc.; and the "amplitude" is the maximum value that the field strength has during any given cycle. Its units would be those of the field in question, i.e., Tesla or Gauss for the magnetic component of an electromagnetic field.

Fig. 3.2 is a graph of the strength of an electromagnetic field (or wave) at some point in space as a function of time. Note the definitions of frequency, period and amplitude in terms of this graph.

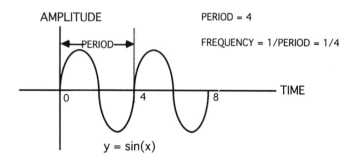

FIG. 3.2- GRAPH OF ELECTROMAGNETIC FIELD vs. TIME–A SINE CURVE

Now an "electromagnetic" wave, as we have described above, can also be called a "radiofrequency" wave. This is an apt term, because all waves have a frequency, and since they are propagated, they can be thought of as **radiating** through space. Furthermore, a "pulse" in general, can be thought of as an extremely brief physical phenomenon. This brings us to the definition of a radiofrequency pulse:

> A **radiofrequency pulse (or RF pulse)** is an electromagnetic wave that results from the brief application of an alternating electric current.

Now let us return to our magnetic resonance scanner. We left the patient at the end of chapter 2 in the magnet with a single vertically oriented vector representing the sum of all the aligned hydrogen MDM vectors. (Actually, there are other species of MDM's that are also aligned, but at this point, we are considering only hydrogen nuclei.)

Axis Conventions

Let us establish the following conventions regarding the relationship of the spatial axes to the patient. The "z axis" runs longitudinally from head to foot; the "x axis" runs from right to left; and the "y axis" runs from front to back.

Hence the axial planes are x-y planes, sagittal planes are y-z planes, and coronal planes are x-z planes (fig. 3.3). These definitions will apply for the remainder of this text.

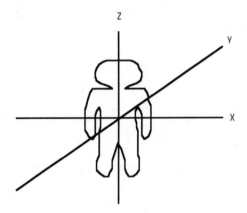

FIG. 3.3- AXIS CONVENTIONS

Perturbance of the M Vector

Using the above terminology, the M vector runs parallel to the z axis. We now "bombard" the patient with a radiofrequency pulse in such a fashion that we cause the M vector to "tip" towards the x-y plane. Actually, the M vector does not simply tip over, it **spirals** its way down such that the head of the vector "draws" a beehive (fig. 3.4). The path that it traces is similar to a road that winds down a mountain from its top to its base.

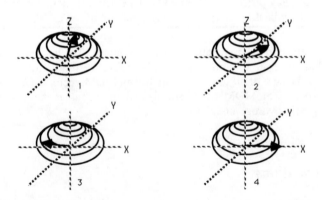

FIG. 3.4- SUCCESSIVE "SNAPSHOTS" OF SPIRALING M VECTOR

This complex motion is really the resultant of two component motions: (1) precession around the z axis, and (2) a tipping motion from the vertical to the horizontal position (i.e., from a position parallel to the z axis to the x-y plane). It seems intuitive that if we "add" these two component movements of the M vector, we will obtain the spiral motion described above (fig. 3.5). In this figure, the second component is shown rotating in the x-z plane around the y axis.

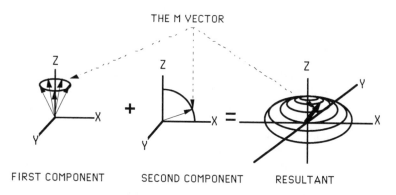

THE M VECTOR

FIRST COMPONENT   SECOND COMPONENT   RESULTANT

FIG. 3.5- TWO PRECESSION COMPONENTS OF THE SPIRAL MOTION OF M

Rotating Frame of Reference

Many texts on this subject make use of the concept of a "rotating frame of reference", which is based on simple Newtonian relativity (not Einsteinian!). For example, if we are standing on the ground watching a merry-go-round with mechanical horses moving up and down, the horses will appear to us to be moving in an undulating fashion-sort of like a sine wave curve. However, if we utilize a rotating frame of reference, that is, if we stand on the moving merry-go-round and rotate with the system, then the horses will appear to be simply moving up and down. We can think of the undulating motion of the horses observed from the ground as consisting of two component motions: (1) the rotation of the merry-go-round, and (2) the up and down displacement of the horses. This is exactly analogous to the magnetic resonance situation. By invoking the rotating frame of reference, we spin around with the precessing M vector, and under those circumstances, the vector simply appears to tip over onto its side.

Now remember that we said that the RF pulse bombards the patient in a certain "fashion". What that means is that the vector direction of the magnetic field component of the RF pulse must be perpendicular to the direction of the main magnetic field of the scanner. Note that we are not talking about the direction of the **propagation** of the field (or wave); the wave propagation of the field occurs in all directions from a point in space. What we **are** talking about is the vector direction of the field (which is related to the direction of the force that a magnetizable substance would experience when it is within the field) regardless of how the field is spreading through space.

Now let us examine a little more carefully the two components of the spiraling M vector. The rotational component around the z axis is due to the fact that the M vector begins to precess when the RF pulse is applied. In chapter 2, we stated that all the individual hydrogen MDM's were precessing around the z axis when the patient is placed in the external magnetic field. We also said that there is a resultant vector (M) which represents the sum of the MDM vectors. However, before the application of the RF pulse, the M vector is **not** precessing (even though the individual MDM's **are** precessing). But once the RF pulse is applied, M itself begins to precess. It is sort of like giving a Foucault pendulum that one little push to get it going. Now the reason that the RF pulse is able to "push" the M vector is related to the second component of the spiral motion.

The second component, as we stated earlier, is the "tipping" motion of the M vector from its z axis position towards the x-y plane. This tipping represents rotation of the M vector around the vector axis of the magnetic field of the RF pulse. This is the "push" effect of the RF pulse. **In other words, the "tipping" motion is precession around an axis perpendicular to the z axis, since the direction of the RF pulse vector is made to be perpendicular to the z axis.** So each component of the spiral motion of the M vector represents precession of M in an axis perpendicular to each of the two magnetic fields in question- the main magnetic field of the scanner and the magnetic field of the RF pulse. The resultant spiral motion of M is the **simultaneous** precession around these two perpendicular directions.

Fig. 3.6a shows several "snapshots" of the spiraling M vector, and fig. 3.6b superimposes on one image these different instants in time. The rotating rectangular plane represents the first component of the motion- precession around the z axis. While the plane rotates around the z axis the vector M rotates downward **in the plane-around the RF pulse vector** (second component of motion). The sum of these two motions produces the spiral movement of M. But since the plane is rotating, the RF pulse vector must also rotate in order for M to precess around it. Hence the RF pulse must actually participate in the rotating frame of reference. In order for it to do that, its frequency must equal that of the rotating plane, which is, of course, the Larmor frequency for the main magnetic field.

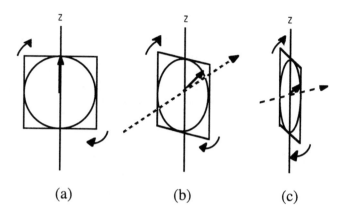

(a)   (b)   (c)

FIG. 3.6a- ROTATING FRAME OF REFERENCE–2 PRECESSION COMPONENTS
The solid straight arrows are the M vector, and the dashed arrows are the RF pulse vector.
As the plane rotates around the z axis, M rotates around the RF pulse vector–2
precessions at right angles to each other. In image (a), the plane faces us *en face* and the
M vector is at 0°. In image (b), the plane has rotated clockwise about 45°, and M has
rotated downward about 45°. In image (c), the plane has rotated about 70° and M has
also rotated about 70°. This process results in M tracing a 3-D spiral.

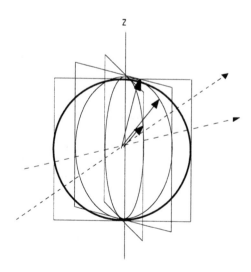

FIG. 3.6b- SUPERIMPOSITION OF THE THREE POINTS IN TIME IN FIG. 3.6a

Resonance

Therefore in order to "tip" or perturb the M vector, the frequency of the RF pulse must equal the Larmor frequency of whatever species of MDM that we wish to affect. This is the concept of **resonance**, and this is how we select the hydrogen MDM over all the various species of precessing MDM's: we simply tune the frequency of the RF pulse to the Larmor frequency of the hydrogen nucleus for the given main magnetic field. And we determine the "resonant frequency", i.e., the frequency necessary to perturb the hydrogen M vector- by applying the Larmor equation: multiply the gyro magnetic ratio of hydrogen times the strength of the main magnetic field in Tesla. If we had wished to perturb the vectors of ^{14}N or ^{31}P, we would simply substitute their gyro magnetic ratios into the Larmor equation to determine their resonant frequencies. The concept of magnetic resonance is analogous to singing into a jar or bowl: if the pitch (frequency) of our voice is just right, the jar will respond by vibrating (resonating).

Note that the precession frequency of the rotation around the RF pulse vector is several orders of magnitude less than the frequency around the z axis. This is because the strength of the magnetic field of the RF pulse is several orders of magnitude less than the strength of the main external magnetic field (remember that the Larmor equation tells us that the precession frequencies are directly proportional to the magnetic field strengths). This means, of course, that we exaggerated things in figs. 3.6 by showing the M vector as rotating **down** the same number of degrees as its **horizontal** rotation. Actually, by the time the M vector would have rotated downward 45 or 70 degrees, it would have already made thousands of complete 360° revolutions in the horizontal plane.

M vs. the Component MDM Vectors

One question that has always plagued residents (and the author) is this: what is happening to the individual MDM vectors while the M vector is spiraling down? The answer is that each one is doing the same thing relative to its own miniature z axis. It is as if the large "beehive" for the M vector contains numerous tiny "beehives" (fig. 3.7). Remember that **prior** to application of the RF pulse, the individual MDM vectors are **not** doing the same thing as the M vector, for the former are precessing, whereas the latter is not.

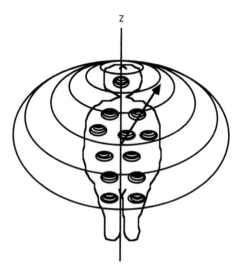

FIG. 3.7- SPIRAL MOTION OF M AND MDM VECTORS
Note that the M vector and the MDM vectors are tracing the same paths relative to each
one's own scale.

This is as much detail as we are going to go into in dealing with the complex
motion of the perturbed M vector. Actually, to have a practical understanding of
how tissue contrast is obtained in MRI (the goal of this section of the book), one
need only understand that the M vector is somehow translated from a vertical
position parallel to the z axis to a horizontal position in the x-y plane. However,
the author has gone into some depth regarding the motion of M because (1) it is
necessary to completely understand the NMR process and (2) many texts and
teachers of the subject have devoted considerable time and effort to explaining
the motion of the M vector, and therefore there is some interest sparked in the
student to come to grips with this topic.

So for the remainder of this text, we will describe the motion of the M vector
under the influence of the RF pulse as simply rotating from its vertical z axis
orientation into the x-y plane (fig. 3.8). In other words, we will make use of the
"rotating frame of reference", as described earlier, and we will imagine ourselves
on a merry-go-round spinning around the z axis at the Larmor frequency of
hydrogen, so that the M vector will appear to us to simply rotate (or flip) from a
vertical to a horizontal position.

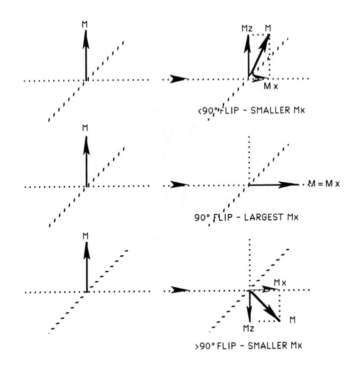

FIG. 3.8- ROTATION OF M FROM Z AXIS TO X-Y PLANE

The Mx and Mz components of M are shown for 3 situations. When M is flipped <90°, Mx (the signal) is not maximal and Mz>0. When M is flipped exactly 90°, M = Mx, Mz = 0 and Mx is maximal. When M is flipped >90°, Mx is again not maximal, and Mz<0.

The Signal and the Mx Vector

Note from fig. 3.8 that if M is "flipped" less than 90° from its z axis orientation, we obtain a **components** of M in both the x and z axes. We will call these vectors the "the Mx and Mz components" of M.

A signal is not a physical entity like a force or a field. A signal is what we *sense* or measure when we detect the presence of an electromagnetic wave. It is the graph of the intensity of an electromagnetic field over time. Signals are combinations of sine and cosine curves (as we saw when we described electromagnetic waves).

There is no measurable signal unless there is a component of M (Mx) in the x-y plane. Since Mx, therefore, represents our signal, the larger the Mx, the greater our signal. Note from fig. 3.8 that the largest signal is obtained when M is flipped exactly 90°. Any flip greater or less than 90° will produce a less than maximal Mx. Of course, when M is flipped 90°, there is **only** an Mx component, and we can think of M as being completely converted to Mx; or we could say that Mx = M and Mz = 0.

So that pretty well completes our coverage of the RF pulse and what it does to the M vector. Here are just a few more details. Remember that the RF pulse is just that: a pulse. It is applied only briefly- perhaps a few milliseconds long.

Controlling the Flip of M

The degree to which M is tipped depends on two factors: (1) the duration of the RF pulse, and (2) the amplitude of the RF pulse. Specifically, the formula that relates the flip angle to these factors is:

$$a = \gamma B_1 t$$

where a is the flip angle, γ is the gyro magnetic ratio, B_1 is the field strength (amplitude) of the RF pulse and t is the time or duration of the pulse. From this formula, we see that the flip angle is directly proportional to the amplitude and the duration of the RF pulse. Hence if, for example, we double the field strength or the duration of the pulse, we double the flip angle, etc. Now, if these factors are just right, M is tipped exactly into the x-y plane. If the duration and/or amplitude is greater than that, then M will be tipped beyond the x-y plane, etc. This concept is utilized in "tuning" the MR scanner to a particular patient prior obtaining a scan.

Motion of M in the X-Y Plane

Note that when M is in the x-y plane, it is simply spinning in that plane like a spinner on a board game. Also, each individual MDM is also spinning in an x-y plane that cuts through its location in the patient. We will have more to say about this in the next chapter, when we discuss relaxation and the signal.

Finally, with regard to the scanner itself, the RF coil is usually the so called "body coil". It surrounds the patient in a similar fashion to the coil of the magnet. We will have more to say about coils in chapter 20.

We now summarize the first two letters ("MR") as follows:

MRR: When the patient is placed in the magnetic field, the MDM's of those nuclei with angular momentum align with the direction of the magnetic field and precess with a frequency directly proportional to the strength of the field. A resultant M vector is produced in the z axis.

MRR: An RF pulse whose magnetic field vector is perpendicular to the z axis is applied, which causes the M vector to spiral down towards the x-y plane. The degree to which this produces an Mx component of M in the x-y plane is the degree to which we obtain an MR signal.

4
Relaxation

We are now ready to embark upon part three of MRR: relaxation. Remember that the RF pulse is exactly that: a *pulse*. It is applied for only a brief period of time, and then it is shut off.

> **Relaxation** is the process that occurs after terminating the RF pulse, in which the physical changes that were caused by the RF pulse return to the state they were in prior to the application of the pulse.

In other words, when we applied the RF pulse, we poured energy into the system (the patient); and as long as the RF pulse was being applied, energy was continually input into the system. However, once the pulse was terminated, the system was left at a higher energy state with nothing to keep it there. And since nature abhors this sort of "unbalanced" state of affairs, it does what it can to rectify the situation and return to "the way things used to be"–at a lower energy state. Of course, when a system goes from a higher to a lower energy state, the extra energy has to go somewhere. This extra energy is released in the form of a signal, which gives us our MR image. Later, we will see that because different tissues have different rates of relaxation, we can obtain different signal intensities, and hence tissue contrast.

T1 and T2 Components of Relaxation

Now let us look more in depth at this relaxation process. Recall that before we applied the RF pulse, we had a vertically oriented M vector (in the z axis), and if we apply the pulse so as to obtain a maximum signal, then we convert the vertical M vector into a horizontal Mx vector. Hence we can understand relaxation as the process by which the horizontal Mx vector reverts back to the vertical M vector. We can consider this deconversion process to be composed of two component processes: (1) re-growth of Mz along the z axis; and (2) decay of Mx in the x-y plane (fig. 4.1).

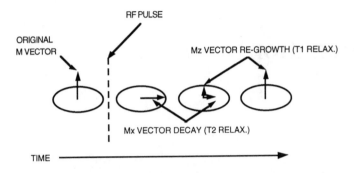

FIG. 4.1- SNAPSHOTS IN TIME OF THE T1 AND T2 COMPONENTS
OF RELAXATION

Re-growth of Mz along the z axis is known as "T1 relaxation", and decay of Mx in the x-y plane is known as "T2 relaxation". These two components of relaxation proceed at different rates depending on the nature of the tissue. The terms "T1" and "T2" are time constants that refer to how long it takes the Mz vector to re-polarize and the Mx vector to decay respectively.[*]   Hence, each tissue has its own T1 and T2 constants.

We will now study T1 in greater depth. However, we will have to wait until chapter 6 to really understand the nature of T2, since it depends on equipment parameters, which we will not discuss in this chapter.

T1 Curves

T1 relaxation curves are graphs that show the strength of the Mz vector as a function of time from the moment that the RF pulse is terminated. This means that the magnitude of the Mz vector is plotted vertically, and time is plotted horizontally. Because of the nature of T1 relaxation, as described above, these curves start at time t=0 (right at the termination of the RF pulse) and magnitude=0, and they steadily increase in intensity over time. They eventually level off as the Mz vector approaches the original strength that it had prior to the RF pulse. As it reaches this point, it approaches complete re-polarization or RECOVERY. Typical T1 relaxation curves are illustrated below in fig. 4.2.

Note that from the graph in fig. 4.2, we can see that water will take a long time to recover its longitudinal or z-axis vector and therefore will have a long T1 constant; whereas fat recovers very rapidly and hence has a relatively short T1 constant.

---

[*] These will be more precisely defined in chapter 5.

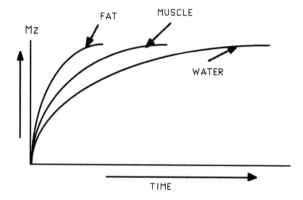

FIG. 4.2- T1 CURVES: Mz MAGNITUDE vs. TIME

It is also the case that a given substance has a longer T1 constant when it is experiencing magnetic resonance in a stronger magnetic field. However, this is not a linear function, as we saw in the case of the Larmor equation, i.e., if we double the field strength, we do not double the T1 constant, even though it does increase.

We have now completed our basic exposition of the three components of the magnetic resonance process **M**agnetic field, **R**F pulse, and **R**elaxation. In the next several chapters, we will see how we can manipulate this process to make our images reflect the fact that different tissues have different T1 and T2 time constants. We will also get a more in-depth understanding of what T2 really is.

We now summarize the first two chapters as follows:

<u>**M**</u>**RR**: When the patient is placed in the magnetic field, the MDM's of those nuclei with angular momentum align with the direction of the magnetic field and precess with a frequency directly proportional to the strength of the field. A resultant M vector is produced in the z axis.

M<u>**R**</u>**R**: An RF pulse whose magnetic field vector is perpendicular to the z axis is applied, which causes the M vector to spiral down towards the x-y plane. The degree to which this produces an Mx component of M in the x-y plane is the degree to which we obtain an MR signal.

MR<u>**R**</u>: The RF pulse is terminated, and the Mx vector in the x-y plane decays and the Mz vector in the z axis re-polarizes as the T1 and T2 components of relaxation simultaneously occur. **As Mx decays, the MR signal decays.**

5
Pulse Cycles, Pulse Sequences, and Tissue Contrast

In order to create an image in space, steps 2 and 3 of **MRR** must be repeated multiple times. That is, the RF pulse must be applied over and over with relaxation and signal measurement occurring after each application of the pulse. The number of such repetitions is usually on the order of 128 or 256 (or some other multiple of 64). Therefore, it is necessary to obtain 128 or 256 signal samples in order to form our image. We are getting a little ahead of ourselves, for this is really the meat of Section II of this book-the image in space. However, to understand how we get tissue contrast, we must be aware that the RF pulse must be repeated many times to produce an image.

We now need two definitions:

A **pulse cycle** is a *repeating* unit which is composed of a series of one or more radio frequency pulses with a measurement of one or more MR signals.

A **pulse sequence** is a series of pulse cycles.

TR and TE

Fig. 5.1 is a simple diagram illustrating a small segment of a chain of multiple RF pulses.

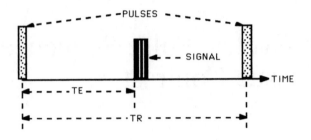

FIG. 5.1- SCHEMATIC DIAGRAM OF A PULSE CYCLE

In this figure, each dot filled rectangle represents a simple RF pulse. The pulse cycle is the unit which is composed of the left sided RF pulse and the signal (line filled rectangle). The right sided RF pulse is the beginning of the next pulse cycle. This is a very simple pulse cycle. Later, we will discuss the *spin-echo* pulse cycle, which contains multiple RF pulses as well as multiple signal measurements.

From fig. 5.1, we obtain two additional definitions:

> **TR** is the time interval between two successive pulse cycles. It is usually measured in milliseconds.

"TR" stands for "Time to Repeat", for it represents the time between pulse cycle repetitions.

> **TE** is the time interval from one pulse (or series of pulses in a more complicated pulse cycle) to the measurement of the MR signal. It is also usually measured in milliseconds.

"TE" stands for "Time to Echo". We stated earlier that the application of the RF pulse causes energy to be input into the patient. The measurement of the signal constitutes the reflection or *echo* of this energy back to us.

The two terms "pulse cycle" and "pulse sequence" are the author's own definitions. The existing literature uses "pulse sequence" to refer to both concepts, and does not distinguish between the two.

Note that there is a fundamental difference between the terms "T1" and "T2" on the one hand, and "TR" and "TE" on the other. T1 and T2 refer to **tissue properties**, whereas TR and TE refer to **equipment parameters**.

T1 and T2 Weighting

Our next major task is to correlate the user defined TR and TE settings with the optimal production of contrast in terms of T1 and T2 relaxation.

Two more definitions:

> A **T1 weighted image** is one in which the intensity contrast between any two tissues in an image is due mainly to the **T1** relaxation properties of the tissues.

> A **T2 weighted image** is one in which the intensity contrast between any two tissues in an image is due mainly to the **T2** relaxation properties of the tissues.

Let us now investigate how we can generate T1 and T2 weighted images by manipulating our pulse cycle parameters: TR and TE.

Fig. 5.2 illustrates the T1 and T2 components of relaxation for two different tissue substances. It is similar to fig. 4.1 in chapter 4 except that it shows **two** examples, each with different T1 and T2 values.

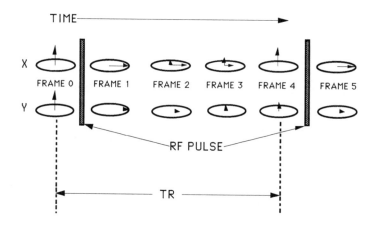

FIG. 5.2- DIFFERENT T1's AND T2's FOR TWO DIFFERENT TISSUES

First, let us consider the relationship of TR to T1. Note that tissue X has a shorter T1 than tissue Y. This is evidenced by the fact that its Mz vector has returned to its original height on frame 4; yet tissue Y's Mz vector is still slightly short of its original height at this point in time. It is taking X less time for its Mz vector to return to its original magnitude, and therefore X's T1 is shorter than Y's. If we choose to repeat the RF pulse right at this time (between frames 4 and 5), as shown in fig. 5.2, then the Mz that will be flipped for X will be taller than the Mz that will be flipped for Y. Therefore, the resulting Mx (horizontal vector) for X will be greater than the Mx for Y, and hence X's signal strength will be greater than Y's immediately after the second RF pulse (frame 5 in fig. 5.2). We can therefore see how different T1 values for different tissues can be responsible for eliciting different signal strengths *with multiple repetitions*. If we were to wait a longer time before applying the second RF pulse (i.e.: use a longer TR), then we would allow more time for Y's slower Mz vector to return to full strength. This would result in equal Mz's, equal Mx's, and equal signal strengths for X and Y. **Hence a longer TR would eliminate the effect of T1 in producing differential signal strengths.**

Next, let us consider the relationship of TE to T2. Note from fig. 5.2 that X's T2 is longer than Y's. This is evidenced from frame 3, where there is still some Mx component for tissue X, but no Mx component for Y. Hence it is taking X longer for its Mx vector to decay, and therefore X's T2 is greater than Y's. If we were to measure our signal at the time of frame 2, for example, then we would record a signal difference corresponding to the two different Mx vector lengths. Hence we see how different tissue T2's result in different signal strengths. However, if we shorten the time we wait to measure the signal (i.e.: use a shorter TE), then we "catch" the Mx vectors before they have a chance to decay, and hence they would be equal (frame 1). **Hence, short TE's eliminate the effect of T2 in producing differential signal strengths.**

So now, we can see how we can manipulate TR and TE to produce T1 and T2 weighted images:

> To produce a **T1 weighted image**, we use a short TE to eliminate the effect of T2 and a short TR in order *not* to eliminate the effect of T1.

> To produce a **T2 weighted image**, we use a long TR to eliminate the effect of T1 and a long TE in order *not* to eliminate the effect of T2.

This can all be easily remembered by a simple silly memory device: "**2**" is greater than "**1**", so **T2** weighted images require greater (longer) TR and TE parameters than **T1** weighted images.

Balanced (Spin Density) Scans

In the next chapter, we will discuss the spin-echo pulse cycle, and we will see that in addition to what was discussed above, most MR scans include an image acquisition with a **long** TR and a **short** TE. Since the long TR cancels the effects of T1 relaxation, and the short TE cancels the effects of T2 relaxation, these images are essentially neither T1 nor T2 weighted. The only factor that is left to influence the contrast of the image is the number of hydrogen nuclei per mm^3. These scans used to be called "proton density" scans. However, we do not image all protons- only hydrogen nuclei. Therefore, it may be more appropriate to use the terms "spin density", "balanced" or "intermediate" scans. So we arrive at yet another definition:

> To produce a **balanced** or **spin density** image, we use a long TR to eliminate the effect of T1 and a short TE to eliminate the effect of T2

In general, a TR greater than 1500 ms , and a TE greater than 40 ms are considered long. Usually, one finds T1 weighted images acquired with TR approximately 500 ms and TE approximately 20 ms; T2 weighted images with TR approximately 2000 ms and TE approximately 80 ms; and balanced images with TR approximately 2000 and TE approximately 20.

It is important to realize that the terms "T1 weighted" and "T2 weighted" cannot be rigidly defined. We cannot draw a line at a certain TR and TE value to differentiate T1 from T2 weighted images. Rather, there is a smooth spectrum from T1 to T2 weighted images. However, that does not lessen the usefulness of these terms as long as we confine ourselves to the two ends of the spectrum. The visible color spectrum flows smoothly from red to ultraviolet making it virtually impossible to "split" one color from another, and yet it makes perfect sense when we refer to colors such as blue and red. Also, TR's are never long enough, and TE's are never short enough to completely eliminate T1 and T2 effects. Hence a given pulse cycle may be relatively more balanced than another.

It is important to point out that the term "T2 weighting", specifically, makes the most sense when it is applied to spin-echo pulse sequences, which will be considered in the next chapter.

6
T2 and the Spin-Echo Pulse Cycle

In preceding chapters, we glibly referred to the T2 decay of the Mx vector after application of the RF pulse. Actually, we oversimplified the case in order not to obscure the understanding of the relationship of T1 and T2 to TR and TE. But now, it is time to delve more deeply into what T2 actually is.

Graph of MR Signal–Free Induction Decay (FID)

Let us begin by looking at exactly what the MR signal is. Remember from chapter 3 that the RF pulse is an electromagnetic wave, which can be described by a mathematical sine curve. Therefore, the MR signal, which is the patient's *reflection* of that RF pulse, must also be a sine curve. However, since Mx, which represents the MR signal, is decaying, the amplitude of the sine curve must also be decaying. Fig. 6.1 illustrates a simple MR signal.

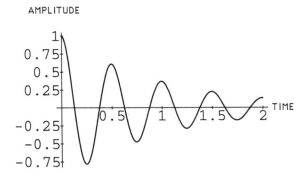

FIG. 6.1- TYPICAL SIMPLE MR SIGNAL

Envelopes of the Signal

Note that the curve is a sort of sine wave with gradually decreasing amplitudes. This signal is known as an "FID" or "free induction decay" signal. Now if we connect the peak positive and peak negative amplitudes of this signal, then we produce the "envelopes" of the curve (fig. 6.2).

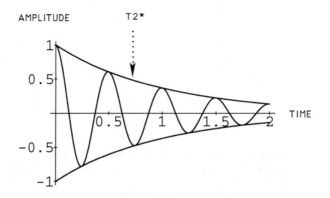

FIG. 6.2- ENVELOPES OF THE FID SIGNAL
The envelopes are the smooth curves joining the peaks of the sine wave. T2* is the upper envelope.

We see from fig. 6.2 that we can describe the essence of the signal by referring to its envelopes, particularly its *positive* envelope.

T2*

Now in previous chapters, we implied that the T2 curve of a tissue was the positive envelope of its FID signal. In other words, we implied that the decay of the Mx vector was "T2 decay". Actually, this is not strictly correct. We cannot obtain T2 decay by simply flipping the M vector into the x-y plane. Simple free induction decay is not T2 decay. Free induction decay proceeds much more rapidly than the true T2 decay, and the positive envelope of the FID signal is more accurately termed the **T2*** curve, as illustrated in fig. 6.2. Hence, what we had been calling "T2 decay" was actually T2* decay.

Concept of Phase

In order to understand true T2, we need to know what causes the FID signal to decay, and in order to do that, we must first understand what "phase" is.

The concept of phase applies only to cyclical processes. This is of fundamental importance, for it makes no sense to speak of the phase of a process unless that process is cycling or repeating its events periodically.

> The **phase** of a process relates a point in its cycle to a point in time. If two cyclic processes are in phase at some point in time, then each of the two processes will be doing the same thing, i.e., each process will be at the same point in its cycle.

One-handed clocks provide the best example illustrating the concept of phase. A cycle on such a clock consists of one rotation of its hand 360 degrees. Now consider two such clocks. They are in phase whenever their hands are pointing at exactly the same angle, i.e., whenever they register the same time. If the hands of the two clocks are spinning at the same rate and are in phase, then they will **always** be in phase as long as they are spinning at the same rate. If the hands of the clocks are **not** in phase, but they are spinning at the same rate, then they will **never** be in phase as long as their rates of spin are the same. If one clock spins twice as fast as the other, then they will be in phase for a brief moment with every revolution of the faster clock, etc. This is illustrated in fig. 6.3 below.

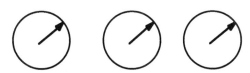

THREE ONE HANDED CLOCKS IN PHASE

THREE ONE HANDED CLOCKS OUT OF PHASE

FIG. 6.3- DEMONSTRATION OF IN PHASE AND OUT OF PHASE

Note that we can represent any cyclic event with a one-handed clock. For example, the cardiac cycle (note the term "cycle") can be represented with end-diastole at 12:00 and end-systole at 6:00, and other events such as valve openings, etc., can be appropriately positioned around the clock. We will develop a simple mathematical concept for phase later in the text.

Phase and the MR Signal

Now that we understand what phase is, we are in a better position to understand why tipping the M vector into the x-y plane produces a signal. The many proton magnetic field vectors can all be considered spinning or precessing as if each one were a one-handed clock. Each precessing vector describes or "draws" a circle just like the one-handed clocks.

Before the application of the RF pulse, the proton magnetic vectors are essentially vertically aligned and are precessing at the Larmor frequency. Each tiny proton magnetic vector (MDM) can be thought of as eliciting its own tiny signal by virtue of its precession motion. However, even though they are all precessing at the same rate, they are **not in phase**, i.e., like the one-handed clocks, they are all spinning at the same rate, but they are not set at the same time. For this reason, their individual signals are not additive but tend to cancel each other out. However, when the RF pulse is applied, all these vectors are forced to be in phase, and hence their individual micro-signals are additive and will yield a resultant signal in the x-y plane.

Dephasing and the MR Signal

Therefore, it follows that the decay of the Mx vector (the T2* curve) is essentially due to **dephasing** of the individual MDM vectors.

Now there are two basic causes for the dephasing of the MDM vectors, and we will consider each one in turn.

(1) Magnetic Field Inhomogeneity (External Magnetic Effects)

Because the main magnetic field is not perfectly uniform, different proton vectors will be precessing at slightly different rates (remember the Larmor equation: the precession frequency is directly proportional to the magnetic field strength). Considering our clock examples of phase, we can see that some precessing MDM's will therefore get out of phase with others. This lack of magnetic field uniformity is one of the two main physical causes for dephasing and hence decay of the Mx vector. We will see later that of the two causes, this is the **correctable** one, and its correction results in the generation of true T2 relaxation from T2* relaxation.

(2) Spin-Spin Interactions (Internal Magnetic Effects)

The second cause of dephasing of the Mx vector is due to the fact that different protons are affected by different neighboring atoms. This affects their individual MDM vector precession rates, and hence dephasing occurs.

We can think of the two causes of dephasing as external and internal magnetic field inhomogeneity.

Rephasing the MR Signal–180° Re-focusing Pulse

As we stated earlier, we can produce true T2 relaxation only if we "correct" the effects of the uneven external magnetic field. How do we do this? Well, if we can in some way reverse the process that is taking place as the MDM's dephase, then we will accomplish our goal. Here is how it is done.

Consider our clock analogy. Let two different one-handed clocks represent two precessing Mx vectors. They are in phase immediately after the 90° pulse (i.e., they register the same time and are proceeding at the same rate). But because of field inhomogeneity, they begin to dephase, i.e., one of the clocks begins to lose time with respect to the other. After a certain period of time t, there is a certain differential time reading on the two clocks. Now, suppose that we cause the two clocks to instantly reverse and proceed in counter-clockwise directions. If we now wait the same amount of time t that it took for the two clocks to get out of phase, then they will return to being in phase (i.e., reading the same time) at time 2t. This is because it will take each of the two clocks exactly the same amount of time to return to the point they were at before they got out of phase. Analogy: if each of several families begins a car trip at exactly the same time, it does not matter what speed they go, for if they all turn 180° around at the same time and proceed at the same speeds, they will all return home at the same time. The faster car has a longer distance to return, and the slower car has a shorter distance to return, so if they maintain the same speeds after turning around, they will return to where they started at the same time.

The mechanism of reversal is accomplished by using a 180° RF pulse which follows the 90° RF pulse (fig. 6.4). The 180° pulse reverses the polarity of the Mx vectors. This causes the effects of the non-homogeneous field to operate in the reverse direction with respect to the Mx vectors.

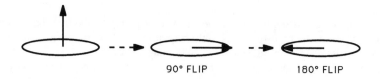

FIG. 6.4- Mx VECTOR FLIPS DURING SPIN-ECHO PULSE CYCLE

The Spin-Echo Pulse Cycle

The important concept here is that the time it takes the vectors to get out of phase must equal the time it takes them to return to phase. The time from the 90° pulse to the 180° pulse must equal the time from the 180° pulse to the measurement of the signal. What we are describing here is the spin-echo pulse cycle:

A **spin-echo pulse cycle** consists of a 90° RF pulse followed by one or more 180° RF pulses, where a signal is measured after each 180° pulse. The time interval from the 90° pulse to the first 180° pulse must equal the time interval from the first 180° pulse to the first signal measurement; and for a second echo in the pulse cycle, the time interval from the first signal measurement to the second 180° pulse must equal the time interval from the second 180° pulse to the second signal measurement.

When a spin-echo pulse cycle contains more than one signal measurement, it is usually called a "multiple echo" (or "multi-echo") pulse cycle.

Fig. 6.5 shows a diagrammatic example of a double echo spin-echo. Note how there are **two** signal measurements, and therefore **two** TE's and **two** 180° pulses. Note also how the 180° pulses "bisect" the time interval between successive signal measurements (or between the first measurement and the 90° pulse), as described above.

Nearly every MR scan makes use of at least one spin-echo pulse sequence, and more specifically, the **double echo** spin-echo is still probably the work-horse of the clinical MR imaging world. A double echo is usually obtained with a long TR (usually around 2000 ms) and two echoes one with a short TE (usually around 20 ms) and one with a long TE (usually around 80 ms). Thus one obtains two sets of images: one with a long TR and a long TE, and the other with a long TR and a short TE. The long TR, **long** TE images are, of course T2 weighted; and the long TR, **short** TE are *balanced* images, as we have defined earlier.

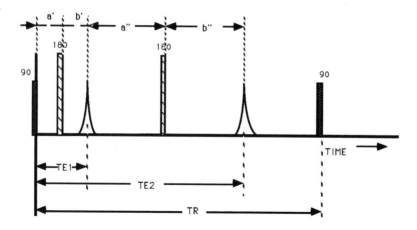

FIG. 6.5- DOUBLE ECHO SPIN-ECHO–NOTE: a'=b' and a"=b"
The clear curved triangles represent the signal measurements. This pulse cycle consists
of a 90° pulse followed by two 180° pulses (and, of course, two signal measurements).

The True T2 Curve

Now, we are ready to understand what the true T2 curve is, in light of the spin-echo pulse cycle. Fig. 6.6 below shows both the T2 and the T2* curves on the same coordinate axes. Note that as we indicated earlier, the T2* curve shows an immediate rapid decay (FID). If there were no 180° pulse, this would be the end of our signal for this cycle. However, because of the 180° pulses, the signal strength is re-instated, reaching a maximum at a time equal to twice the interval from the 90° pulse (or last echo) to the 180° pulse. Note also that each rejuvenation of the signal yields a peak intensity that is somewhat less than the previous one. We can never **completely** restore the signal because of the other contribution of dephasing: spin-spin interactions. It is like a bouncing ball, which never bounces as high as the last bounce because of friction. In other words, the 180° pulse eliminates the effects of the inhomogeneous magnetic field and allows decay to be a function of spin-spin interactions only. This is true T2 decay. We can think of the 180° pulse as a "re-focusing" pulse, which eliminates external "artifactual" causes of dephasing and allows only the tissue characteristics, i.e., internal magnetic field inhomogeneities, to prevail as the main dephasing cause.

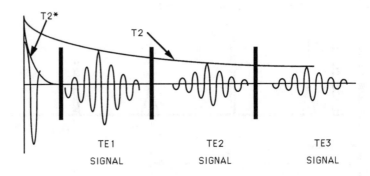

FIG. 6.6- THE TRUE T2 CURVE

The y axis is signal intensity, and the x axis is time for the T2* curve, but **TE** for the true T2 curve. The signals at TE1, TE2 and TE3 represent continuation of the T2* curve in real time. The dark vertical bars represent the 180° re-focusing pulses.

Now, if we connect the peaks of the re-focused or rejuvenated signals caused by the 180° pulses, then we will obtain a curve envelope which represents the true T2 curve for that tissue in that pulse cycle. It is important to realize that unlike the T2* curve, the T2 curve is **not** a "real time" curve; that is, it is not a graph of signal intensity over real time, because if one considers a point in time **between** the re-focused signals, there would be very little or no signal at all, and yet the T2 envelope curve is certainly not zero. Therefore, the T2 curve is a graph of the signal intensity vs. **TE** for a given tissue with a given TR. It is not a graph of the signal intensity vs. **time**. (T2* is a graph of intensity vs. real time.) The T2 curve shows us what signal intensity we *WOULD* get if we imaged that particular tissue with a spin-echo utilizing that particular TR and a selected TE. This, of course assumes that the TE and the 180° pulses will be properly coordinated in time, as described above. **Each point on the T2 curve can be obtained by applying an initial 90° pulse, applying a 180° pulse at any time (t, for example) and then measuring the signal intensity at time 2t. Simply plot this point on the graph with 2t as the x coordinate and the signal intensity as the y coordinate.**

T2 Curves for Different Tissues for Long TR's

We can mathematically determine the T2 curve for any tissue, given TR and the tissue's T1 and T2 for the magnetic field strength being used. This is done by solving a partial differential equation known as the "Bloch equation". The calculus manipulations necessary to derive this formula are beyond the scope of this text (as well as the author), but the formula itself is relatively simple and is listed below.* Fig. 6.7 uses this formula to plot T2 curves for fat, muscle, water and tumor (prostate carcinoma) for a TR of 2000 ms in a 1.5T magnet. The T1 and T2 values for these tissues were obtained from experimental determinations done by prior investigators.

T1 and T2 Constants

It should be pointed out at this time that T1 and T2 do not actually represent the total time it takes either for M to reconstitute or for Mx to decay. This is because it would be difficult to define those end points. T1 is the time it takes for Mz to return to approximately 63% of its original value; and T2 is the time it takes for Mx to diminish to approximately 37% of its initial value.**

TR=2000 (1.5T)

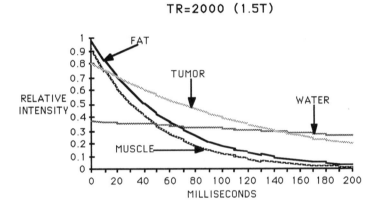

FIG. 6.7- T2 CURVES OF FAT, MUSCLE, WATER AND TUMOR FOR TR=2000 IN A 1.5 TESLA MAGNET

Note that we get the greatest contrast (i.e., the greatest signal *difference*) between tumor and either muscle or fat if we use a TE around 100 ms. Since both TR and TE are relatively long, we could call this a T2 weighted pulse sequence. In general, there is good contrast delineation between tumors and other tissues when T2 weighted pulse sequences are used.

---

* $I = r(1 - e^{-TR/T1}) e^{-TE/T2}$; where I is the resulting signal intensity, r is the proton or spin density, e is the natural base, and TR, TE, T1 and T2 are as discussed above.
** More precisely, the .63 number is really 1-1/e, and the .37 number is 1/e, where e is the natural base. Hence T1 is **exactly** defined as the time it takes for B0 to return to (1-1/e) times its original magnitude; and T2 is **exactly** defined as the time it takes for B1 to decay to 1/e times its initial value.

Note again that when a short TE is used (20 ms), water has the lowest signal of the four; and when a long TE is used (160 ms), water has the highest signal. This explains why on an MR brain scan, the ventricles and cisterns are dark on the balanced images, but bright on the T2 weighted images. (The T2 curve for CSF crosses the T2 curve for brain tissue similar to the way water crosses muscle and fat in the above example.)

Finally, note that the longer the TE, the lower all of the signals are, and therefore, the poorer the quality of the image statistically. This explains why heavily T2 weighted images often appear more noisy or grainy than other images. Along these same considerations, long TR's give us greater signals than short TR's, because we allow Mz to more completely re-polarize, and when it is subsequently "flipped", we get a higher initial signal (c.f. chapter 4). Also, short TE's yield larger signals than long TE's, because Mx is not given the time to decay. This implies that balanced sequences (long TR and short TE) give us images with the most signal strength and hence the least graininess or mottle.

T2 Curves for Different Tissues for Short TR's

Fig. 6.8 below is exactly like fig. 6.7 except that a short TR of 500 ms was used instead of 2000 ms.

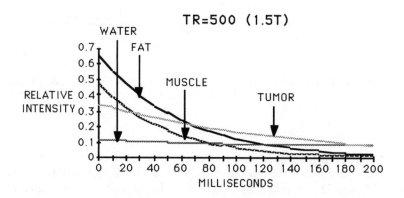

FIG. 6.8- T2 CURVES FOR FAT, MUSCLE WATER AND TUMOR FOR TR=500 IN A 1.5 TESLA MAGNET

Note that the greatest separation between signal magnitudes (esp. between fat, muscle and water), i.e., is obtained when we use very short TE's. And likewise, as we use longer and longer TE's, the T2 curves for the tissues become more and more bunched together with a consequent loss in contrast. Also, of course, the longer the TE, the less the over all signal strength. Hence we have three good reasons why we should try to use as short a TE as possible to obtain T1 weighted images:

(1) Short TE's cancel the T2 effects (from chapter 4).

(2) Short TE's usually yield greater contrast.

(3) Short TE's yield greater signal strength.

SECTION II
The Image in Space

7
Gradients

Now that we have learned from Section I of this book how and why different tissues appear as different intensities, we will concentrate on understanding how these different intensities are arranged in space to produce an image. There are a number of ways of doing this, but in this section, we will be concerned only with the most widely used method: two dimensional Fourier transform ("2DFT") reconstruction.

A magnetic resonance imaging acquisition consists of a set of planar images through some volume of tissue-the brain, for example. Each plane (or slice) contains a two dimensional image which is composed of intensities located on this plane with the use of two coordinates. Hence two coordinate axes are necessary to portray the image on each plane. Since there are multiple planes situated at different levels, a third axis is necessary to locate the position of each plane. Hence, a magnetic resonance imaging acquisition is a three dimensional phenomenon and requires three coordinate axes.

The code or language that MRI uses to locate points on these three axes is in terms of the "gradient". We will now define "gradient" in two ways: linguistically and mathematically:

LINGUISTIC: A **gradient** is a quantitative change in some variable that occurs from one point in space to another.

The change is virtually always a continuous one. A slope of a hill represents a gradient because it is a change in height that occurs as we move along a certain direction on the hill. Likewise, if a force or pressure varies from one point to another, then we have a force or pressure gradient.

MATHEMATICAL: a gradient is the slope of a linear function: it is **m** in the equation y = **mx** *.

It is important to understand the gradient as a quantity, for that will help to understand how the phase encoding gradient is gradually increased (to be discussed later).

In magnetic resonance imaging, we use magnetic field gradients to produce an image. This simply means that the magnetic field magnitude varies from one point in space to another. What we are referring to here is the main external magnetic field. When we impose a gradient on it, we cause this field strength to vary (slightly) along a certain line, rather than maintaining a constant 1.5T at all points in the field. And in fact, this variation in field strength is linear. With regard to our mathematical definition of gradient, a magnetic field gradient is a numerical value which is the slope of a straight line graph representing the variation of the magnetic field from one point to another. Since, as we stated earlier, it takes three coordinates to localize a point in space, we need three magnetic field gradients oriented along the three major axes in space. Fig. 7.1a shows the graphs of three different magnetic field gradients: a reference gradient (g), its inverse (-g), and a gradient twice the amplitude of g (2g).

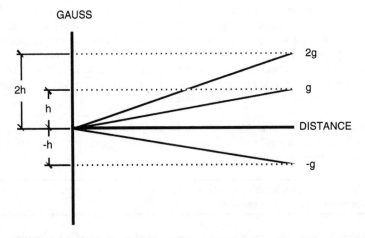

FIG. 7.1a- GRAPHS OF MAGNETIC FIELD STRENGTH (GAUSS) vs. DISTANCE
Note that the 2g gradient is twice the amplitude (slope) of the g gradient, because for any point along the distance axis, its Gauss value is twice that of the g gradient. Also, the -g gradient is the inverse of the g gradient, because for any point on the distance axis its Gauss value is the negative of that of the g gradient.

---

* The usual equation for a straight line is y = mx + b, where m is the slope, and b is the y intercept. The gradient curve is considered to run through the origin, so there is no y intercept, and hence b = 0.

Later on, we will want to diagram the application of gradients along a time axis to show how strong and for how long they are applied. Fig. 7.1b shows how we will do this for the three gradients in fig. 7.1a.*

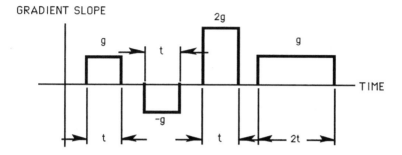

FIG. 7.1b- GRAPHS OF THE GRADIENT SLOPES vs. TIME

The gradients g, 2g, and -g in fig. 7.1a are straight lines, and therefore their slopes are constant. Hence they are shown as horizontal lines on this graph. Note how the first 3 gradients are applied for a time t; whereas the 4th gradient is the g gradient applied for twice that length of time. We will use "bracket" graphs of this sort later when we show how gradients are applied in pulse sequences and how they modify spinning MDM vectors.

Now in order to produce an image, one gradient is used to locate the level of each plane and is known as the "slice select" gradient; and the other two gradients are used to locate points of intensity within each plane. They are called the "frequency" and "phase encoding" gradients. These terms will become more clear as we proceed. For most of the remainder of this text, the slice select gradient will be in the z axis, and the frequency and phase encoding gradients will be in the x and y axes respectively (as these axes have been defined in chapter 3). Note that in fig. 7.1a, distance is the z axis for the slice select gradient, the x axis for the frequency gradient and the y axis for the phase encoding gradient. We will now discuss the role each of these gradients plays in creating the image.

---

* For math buffs: these "bracket" gradients are simply the derivatives of the gradient curves (slopes).

8
The Slice Select Gradient

Of the three gradients, we will begin with the slice select gradient. Since it is in the z axis direction, we will call it the "z gradient". The z gradient imposes a gradual change in the main magnetic field from the head to the foot end of the patient. If we graph the z gradient with the magnitude of the magnetic field on the y axis and the position along the long axis of the body on the x axis, then we obtain the straight line shown in the graph in fig. 8.1 below.

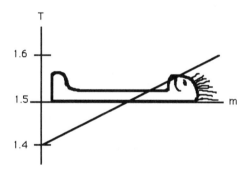

FIG. 8.1- DISTANCE IN METERS vs. MAGNITUDE IN TESLA

Note that the field intensity varies from greater than 1.5T at the head end of the patient to less than 1.5T at the feet end. The 1.5T point would fall somewhere midway between the head and the feet. Actually, in real life, the gradient is much less steep than the .2T difference illustrated in fig. 8.1.

The gradient is achieved by adding a set of coils to the coils that produce the main external magnetic field.

Now recall the Larmor equation. Since the precession frequency of the magnetic dipole moment (MDM) vectors is directly proportional to the magnetic field strength, we can substitute frequency for intensity along the Y axis with a suitable change in scale. In other words, the Larmor equation tells us that to find the frequency of the MDM's, simply multiply the field strength by a constant (the gyro magnetic constant). Hence we can change the y axis of figure 8.1 from field strength (Tesla) to frequency (cycles per second) by multiplying each point along the axis by a constant. This gives us the graph in fig. 8.2.

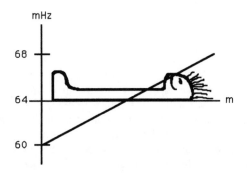

FIG. 8.2- DISTANCE IN METERS vs. FREQUENCY IN MHz

We see, therefore, that the MDM vectors are precessing at different frequencies from one end of the body to the other. Now, remember from chapter 3 that the only proton vectors that are "flipped" by the RF pulse are those whose precession frequency equals the frequency of the RF pulse (resonance). Hence, by selecting a certain RF pulse frequency, we will select a plane in which the proton vectors are to be "flipped" (i.e., we flip only those MDM vectors within that certain plane; no other vectors will be affected by the RF pulse). Hence, we select an image plane. Actually, we do not use a single RF frequency, for that would theoretically yield an "infinitesimally" thin cut. Instead, we use a range of frequencies, which define a finitely thick imaging plane.

Changing Slice Thickness

Note that as a consequence of the above, we can alter the thickness of the image slice in two ways: (1) change the range of frequencies of the RF pulse; and (2) change the slope of the Z gradient. In fig. 8.3, slice **a** is thicker then slice **b** because its RF band width or range of frequencies is greater (the outer pair of horizontal lines spans a larger distance than the inner lines) . In fig. 8.4, slice **a** is thicker because the **gradient** is less steep.

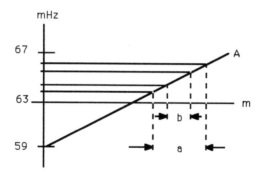

FIG. 8.3- CHANGING SLICE THICKNESS BY VARYING RF FREQUENCY WIDTH
The wider RF pulse (thick horizontal lines) contains frequencies ranging from 64 to 66 MHz; whereas the narrower pulse (thin horizontal lines) contains frequencies from about 64.5 to 65.5 MHz.

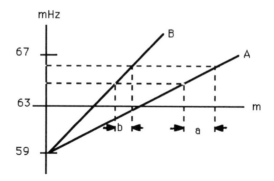

FIG. 8.4- CHANGING SLICE THICKNESS BY VARYING THE GRADIENT STEEPNESS
The RF frequency width remains constant here (dashed horizontal lines). But gradient B is steeper than gradient A, and this causes slice b to be thinner than slice a.

Although we have presented two alternatives for altering the slice thickness, most manufacturers use the method of varying the gradient steepness. Incidentally, because the gradients are steeper for thinner slices, this puts more "work" on the gradients, and this is why you may have encountered limitations in your choice of parameters when you set up a scan with very thin slices.

It is important to point out that the magnetic field gradients are not on all the time. In fact, each is turned on briefly at various points in the pulse cycle. **The z axis or slice select gradient is turned on only during the application of the RF pulses.**

9
Frequency Gradient

So far, we have shown how we select an image plane, which represents only the first of the three coordinates that we must specify. To complete our image, we must understand how the other two orthogonal gradients specify the other two coordinates of each point in a given plane.

The Pixel Grid

We can consider each slice as being composed of a grid of "picture elements" known as "pixels". Each pixel will have its own signal strength.[*] In order to obtain a magnetic resonance image, our goal will be to determine the signal strength for each individual pixel. Now it would be ideal if we could measure the signal in each pixel separately, but that is impossible. The only thing we can measure is the entire composite signal from all the pixels. Hence, the mathematical task is to reconstruct the value of the signal intensity of each individual pixel given the composite signal.

Let us consider a theoretical simplified axial slice of tissue with a 4x4 pixel grid. Let each pixel be associated with a certain signal strength. Fig. 9.1 illustrates this pixel grid. Now if we assign a gray scale to our signal strengths, we obtain the "image" in fig. 9.2.

Sine Functions for Each Pixel

Next, remember from chapter 3 that signals are graphs of electromagnetic field intensity, and that they therefore can be represented by trigonometric sine functions: $I = A\sin(nt)$, where I is the signal intensity, A is the amplitude and n is the frequency. Now we will substitute these sine functions for each pixel in our

---

[*] We will have more to say on the concept of the pixel in a later chapter.

grid, letting each amplitude A equal the corresponding value for that pixel in fig. 9.1., and letting the frequency arbitrarily = 1 for all pixels. This is shown in fig. 9.3. Note that for this discussion, we are not concerned about decay of the signal over time; hence we can use simple sine functions as shown above.

4	3	1	6
8	1	2	7
3	5	2	6
1	4	8	3

FIG. 9.1- SAMPLE TISSUE SLICE WITH 16 PIXELS
Each number represents the relative signal strength for that pixel

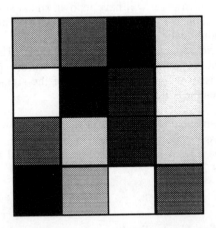

FIG. 9.2- GRAY SCALE IMAGE CORRESPONDING TO THE RELATIVE
SIGNAL STRENGTHS IN FIG. 9.1
Note that according to present day imaging conventions, the brighter pixels correspond to higher signal strengths.

4sin(t)	3sin(t)	sin(t)	6sin(t)
8sin(t)	sin(t)	2sin(t)	7sin(t)
3sin(t)	5sin(t)	2sin(t)	6sin(t)
sin(t)	4sin(t)	8sin(t)	3sin(t)

FIG. 9.3- SINE FUNCTION REPRESENTATION OF EACH PIXEL'S
SIGNAL STRENGTH

Note that the amplitude for each sine function corresponds to the relative signal strength for that pixel in fig. 9.1. Note also that this is prior to the application of a gradient, and therefore the frequencies are all the same: 1.

Application of Frequency Gradient

To distinguish points along the x axis, a magnetic field gradient is applied in the direction of the x axis. This means that the magnitude of the magnetic field will vary from the right side to the left side of the patient (and from right to left on our 4 x 4 pixel grid). Now, remembering the Larmor equation, the precession frequencies of the proton magnetic vectors will also vary from point to point along the x axis.

In our sample tissue slice, this results in four columns of vectors with each column precessing at a different frequency. We will let 1, 2, 3 and 4 represent the frequency for each column from left to right. This is depicted in fig. 9.4. This is what a frequency gradient (often termed "read-out gradient") does.

When the resultant signal is measured, it represents the sum of the signals from each of the 16 pixels. Since the frequency is the same within each column, the sum of the signals in each column can be represented by a single term (that is, we algebraically add the terms in each column): column 1 = 16sin(t); column 2 = 13sin(2t); column 3 = 13sin(3t) and column 4 = 22sin(4t). So the total composite signal equals 16sin(t) + 13sin(2t) + 13sin(3t) + 22sin(4t).

4sin(t)	3sin(2t)	sin(3t)	6sin(4t)
8sin(t)	sin(2t)	2sin(3t)	7sin(4t)
3sin(t)	5sin(2t)	2sin(3t)	6sin(4t)
sin(t)	4sin(2t)	8sin(3t)	3sin(4t)

X GRADIENT ──────────────────➤

FIG. 9.4- SIGNAL GRID DURING APPLICATION OF FREQUENCY GRADIENT
In contrast to fig. 9.3, we are applying a gradient, which causes each column to have a different frequency. The frequencies are represented by the coefficients of t: 1 for column 1, 2 for column 2, 3 for column 3 and 4 for column 4.

Note that just as the z axis gradient is applied only at a certain time (i.e.: when the RF pulse is applied), so it is with the x axis gradient, which is applied **only when the signal is measured**. (Sometimes the frequency gradient is referred to as the "read-out gradient".)

At this point, the machine receives a composite signal consisting of the sum of four sine wave functions, as shown above. We will consider what happens to this signal in more detail later in chapter 12.

Now what we would like the scanner to do at this point is to tell us what the sum of the signal strengths is for each column in the pixel grid using the information from the received signal. However, the MR scanner cannot *immediately* perceive that information from the signal as recorded. The information is there, but it is in a hidden form. It must be extracted by a special technique: **Fourier transformation**. We must use a mathematical device to decode the information encoded in the signal. Since the Fourier transform is so important in the analysis of the signal, we will devote the next chapter to understanding it in terms of simple algebraic and non-mathematical terms.

10
The Fourier Transform

We will eventually show that a Fourier transform is a spectrum. Hence it is necessary to know what a spectrum is.

The Spectrum

Suppose we have 230 students who have taken an examination. We could then describe the results by indicating how many students got each of the different grades from 0 to 100%. Fig. 10.1 below shows a bar graph of just such a situation, where the x axis represents the score, and the y axis indicates how many students got each score. This graph is a form of spectrum. It shows us the distribution of the grades.

A **spectrum** is a distribution graph or curve. A spectrum is also sometimes known as a **profile**.

The Fourier Series

A well-known mathematical theorem tells us that nearly any smooth algebraic function can be represented by an infinite series of sines and cosines. Hence a parabola ($y=x^2$), a diagonal line ($y=x$), or a horizontal line ($y=5$) can all be approximated by a series of trigonometric functions. These are known as "Fourier series", and for a given function $f(x)$, they are written:

$$f(x) = C + a_1\sin(x) + a_2\sin(2x) + a_3\sin(3x) + ... + a_n\sin(nx)$$

$$+ b_1\cos(x) + b_2\cos(2x) + b_3\cos(3x) + ... + b_n\cos(nx).$$

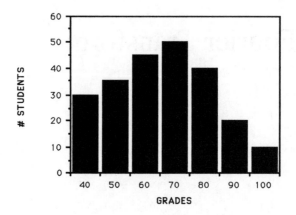

FIG. 10.1- SAMPLE SPECTRUM SHOWING THE DISTRIBUTION OF
GRADES AMONG THE STUDENTS

Note that as n approaches infinity (i.e., as the series is made longer and longer), the series more accurately approximates f(x). Also, the coefficients a_1, a_2, etc. are all determined depending on what f(x) is. Just *how* they are determined involves the application of integral calculus, which we will not go into here.

Recall that the coefficient of the variable within a sine or cosine function represents the frequency. If we examine the Fourier series carefully, we note that each successive sine or cosine term has a higher frequency than the terms before it, i.e., sin(3x) has a higher frequency than sin(2x), etc. Hence, a Fourier series is a sum of sines and cosines of increasing frequency where the coefficients (a_1, a_2, etc.) tell us the amplitude of each frequency component. Hence, we could describe a particular Fourier series by graphing the amplitude for each frequency term or component.

For example, consider the following finite portion of a Fourier series: f(x) = 3sin(x) + 4sin(2x) + 6sin(3x) + 7sin(4x). We could draw a graph in which the frequencies 1, 2, 3 and 4 are plotted on the x axis, and their respective amplitudes 3, 4, 6 and 7 are plotted on the y axis (fig. 10.2). This is a spectrum. Just as the student spectrum showed us how many students got each grade, this curve shows us how much of each frequency is present.

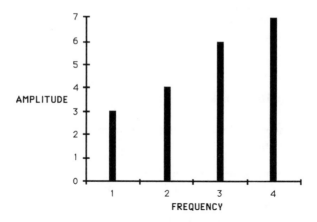

FIG. 10.2- SPECTRUM OF A SAMPLE FOURIER SERIES: A FOURIER
TRANSFORM

Note that the graph of the Fourier spectrum described above consists of discrete
lines or bars at integral frequencies 1, 2, 3 and 4. In other words, it is not
continuous. A Fourier **transform**, on the other hand, **is** a continuous frequency
distribution curve. It is a curve rather than a bar graph. However, because we
will be dealing with sines and cosines as our functions, it turns out that their
Fourier transforms are like bar graphs anyway. In other words, for the purpose
of understanding magnetic resonance signals, we can think of a Fourier
transform as a bar graph spectrum of a Fourier series, as we explained above.

> The **Fourier transform** of a given function can be thought of as the spectrum of
> that function's Fourier series. [*]

Now we stated earlier that every continuous function can be written as a Fourier
series. And since every Fourier series has an associated spectrum, which we can
think of as a Fourier transform, it follows that every continuous function has a
Fourier transform. Now it turns out that the transform of a transform is the
original function. In other words, if the transform of **f** is **F**, then the transform of
F is **f**. So the Fourier transform behaves like a toggle- switching back and forth
between a function and its transform. Later we will see that this property of the
Fourier transform is crucial to the final step of image reconstruction.

In general, the Fourier transform of a given function tells us something about
that function's complexity. If we have a function that represents an image, then

---

[*] According to strict mathematical principles, this is not exactly correct, but the author
believes it will help the reader to better understand the concept of the Fourier transform.

the intricacy of the image will correlate with the amount of high frequency components in the function's Fourier spectrum. If the image is simple, then the Fourier transform (or spectrum) of its function will not contain very many high frequency components.

Fourier Transform of Pixel Grid

Now let us see how we apply the Fourier transform to the composite signal from our sample pixel grid.

We will consider the composite signal formula as a function of the variable t, which we will call "f(t)". Remember that the Fourier transform of a function is a spectrum which plots frequencies on the horizontal axis vs. their amplitudes on the vertical axis. Now the function f(t) is itself composed of sines having amplitudes and frequencies. Therefore, it just so happens that when we apply the Fourier transform to f(t), we obtain a spectrum that plots the frequencies 1, 2, 3 and 4 on the x axis; and the amplitudes 16, 13, 13 and 22 on the y axis (fig. 10.3).[*]

We originally stated that our goal is to specify the signal strength of each pixel in order to create our image. In the above example, the frequencies 1,2,3 and 4 represent the four columns in the 16 pixel grid. Hence, the points (1,16), (2,13), (3,13) and (4,22) on the Fourier transform tell us that the first column has an amplitude of 16, the second column 13, third column 13 and the fourth column 22. Remember that each of these amplitudes represents the sum of the pixel amplitudes in each **column**. Therefore, the Fourier transform of the composite signal gives us the signal strength of each column of pixels.

Hence, we must do more to extract the signal strength of each **individual pixel**. At this point our situation is analogous to a CT image in which only one projection is obtained: in order to complete the slice we need many more projections.

The reader should also note that what we have been describing in this chapter is a *one dimensional* Fourier transform, whereas MR image reconstruction requires a *two* dimensional Fourier transform. However, we must understand the concept of a one dimensional transform before we can go on to higher dimensions.

---

[*] For math lovers only: actually, the spectrum in fig. 10.3 should really be plotted in the complex plane, since the sum of these sine functions is not an even function, and therefore its transform is not real.

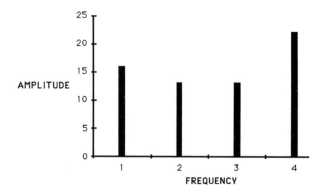

FIG. 10.3- FOURIER TRANSFORM (SPECTRUM) OF COMPOSITE SIGNAL

Rotating Gradients–One Alternative

To obtain the additional information, we could proceed as in CT scanning and create more projections at different angles. We could do this by simply rotating the x gradient around the patient and acquire many sums of amplitudes at different angles. Then we could apply the CT algorithms to reconstruct the image. The problem with this method is that since the x gradient is rotated around the patient, it is critical that the external magnetic field be perfectly uniform. Since this is not practically possible, this method would yield inaccurate reconstructions. The use of phase encoding will be discussed in the next chapter.

11
The Phase Encoding Gradient

The y gradient is applied in the direction perpendicular to the coronal plane. Now it would seem that we could be able to use frequency in this direction just as we did for the x axis. However, if we did that, then we would not be able to uniquely specify whether a given frequency belonged to the x or the y axis, and the computer would get confused and render us an improper image reconstruction. So we must do something else, and in fact, all commercial scanners available today make use of "phase encoding". This rather difficult concept will now be explained in depth.

Remember that as soon as the M vector is "flipped" into the x-y plane, all of the precessing vectors are in phase (chapter 6). Now let us apply a gradient in the y axis for a short period of time during the pulse cycle after the application of the RF pulse. Once again, this means that we are causing the magnetic field magnitude to vary along a certain direction–this time from the front to the back of the patient. Again, because of the Larmor equation, **while the y gradient is on**, each **row** of vectors will precess at a different frequency. Next, we turn the y gradient off. Immediately, the vectors will all precess at the same frequency again. However, now they are no longer in phase, i.e., they are all pointing in different directions as they spin at the same rate.

If we reconsider the one-handed clock analogy, we had all the clocks' hands spinning at the same rate and set to the same time before the application of the y gradient. During the application of the y gradient, each row of clocks perpendicular to the y axis begins to spin at a different rate, so that when the y gradient is terminated, the various rows of clocks are now each set at a different time even though their cycling rate is again equalized.

Another analogy that we can use to represent the situation at this time is to consider different clocks in various time zones around the world. The clocks are all set at different times (i.e., they are not in phase), yet they all keep accurate time (i.e., their hands all rotate at the same frequency). The y gradient is used to set the clocks at different times.

In other words, the y gradient is used to shift the phase of each of the rows of vectors. We can understand phase shifts as **displacements** of the spinning vectors; and those displacements result from different spin frequencies of the vectors. Thus we can think of phase and frequency as analogous to distance and velocity respectively in rate-time problems. If one car drives 50 mph and another drives 100 mph, then after a certain period of time, there will be a certain distance between the two cars. Likewise, if one vector is spinning at 100 Hz, and another is spinning at 200 Hz, then after 1 mS, there will be an angular "distance" between the two vectors. This angle represents a **phase shift** between the two vectors. This leads us to a simple mathematical concept of phase:

If a vector has a constant frequency, then its phase shift over a period of time will be equal to its frequency multiplied by the time, or $\phi = \omega t$ where ϕ is the phase shift, ω is the frequency, and t is time.

And this is just like saying that distance equals rate multiplied by time.

Degrees of Phase Shift per Row

The phase *difference* between rows of vectors is an angular measurement which is equal to 360/n, where n equals the number of rows. In our 16 pixel example, there are four rows, so the phase shift *difference* between rows would be 360/4 or 90 degrees. The gradient is applied in such a fashion that its zero point is approximately at the mid point of the y axis. This has the effect of causing positive phase shifts to one side of the mid-line and negative shifts to the other side. If we number the rows of our 4 x 4 grid, then the mid-line would be between rows 2 and 3. Row 2 would be shifted 90°, and row 1 would be shifted 180°, whereas row 3 would be shifted -90°, and row 4 would be shifted -180°. This is illustrated in fig. 11.1a below.

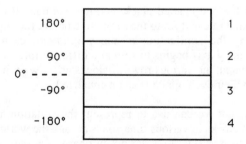

FIG. 11.1a- ROWS OF PHASE SHIFTS: 0 TO 180° UP, AND 0 TO -180° DOWN

Now what we have described so far is not entirely accurate. Remember that a gradient is the slope of a linear function, and if a linear function is to produce a phase shift between rows, then that shift must be the same between any two rows. If we look at fig. 11.1a carefully, then we see that the phase shift between rows 1 and 2 is 90°, whereas the phase shift between rows 2 and 3 is **180°**. Hence we must modify fig. 11.1a by letting 0° represent a row rather than a line between rows. Now if we were to insist upon symmetry to either side of the 0° row, then this would necessitate an odd number of rows (5 rows). But the mathematical algorithms used in commercial scanners for the Fourier transform will not work correctly to yield an image unless there are an even number of rows. Hence we wind up with the situation illustrated in fig. 11.1b, in which the 0° row is offset by one row:

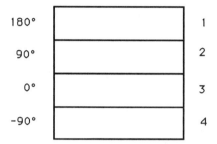

FIG. 11.1b- CORRECTED PHASE SHIFT ROWS

Now, there is exactly 90° phase difference between each row. This also applies to row 4 and row 1. We can see the cyclic nature of this process.

The 0° offset is not nearly as dramatic in a commercial scanner, where there are a minimum of 128 rows, so that there would be 64 rows above and 63 rows below the 0° row.

The above process is called "phase encoding", and it allows us to "mark" the signal with a co-ordinate in the y axis.

Phase Shift in Sine Functions

Let us digress briefly in order to incorporate the concept of *phase* into mathematical notation, which we will need to use in subsequent illustrations. The phase of a sine (or cosine) curve refers to its position on the x axis. If we shift the phase, then we shift the curve either to the right or the left. Fig. 11.2 illustrates two sine curves that differ only in their phase. Algebraically, we express a phase shift by adding a constant to the term within the sine function itself. Consider the curve y=sin(nx+p). Here, p is a term that represents a phase shift, which depends on the value of p. If p is positive, the curve shifts to the left; if it is negative, the curve shifts to the right; if it is zero, there is no shift. Hence, the general algebraic expression for a sine curve is: y=Asin(nx+p), where A=amplitude, n=frequency and p=phase shift. Note that this is consistent with our previous discussions of phase: when we compare two sine curves that differ in phase, the difference in their positions on the x axis reflects the fact that at any point in time, each curve is at a different point in its cycle.

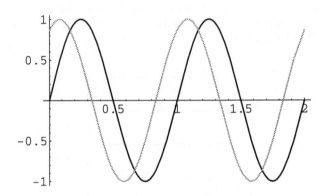

FIG. 11.2- TWO SINE CURVES OF THE SAME FREQUENCY
OUT OF PHASE BY 60°

The darker curve is y = sin(2πx) and the lighter curve is y = sin(2πx+π/3). The lighter curve is shifted to the left with respect to the darker curve by π/3 (60°). Both curves have the same frequency.

Simple Summary of Phase Ideas

At this point, it will be helpful to summarize the three concepts of phase that we have been using in this book:

(1) Two cyclic processes are in phase at a given point in time if they are at the same point in their cycles.

(2) If two sine or cosine functions have the same frequency, then we can mathematically express a phase shift by adding a constant term to the expression within the sine or cosine function.

(3) A phase shift can be mathematically expressed as frequency multiplied by time ($\phi = \omega t$).

Multiple Repetitions to Form the Image

Remember that when we discussed the generation of the MR signal in Section I, we talked about TR–the repetition time. It is necessary that we have a repetition time in order to create enough information to generate an image. It turns out that **the number of repetitions equals the number of rows of vectors in the pixel grid.**[*] For each repetition, the y gradient is applied with an incrementally increasing slope. This means that with each succeeding repetition, the effect of the y gradient is greater than the previous repetition. Let us illustrate this in detail with our 4 x 4 sample pixel grid.

Since it is a 4 x 4 grid, there are four phase encoded rows of vectors and four repetitions. For the first "repetition", no phase encoding gradient is used (i.e.: the phase shift is 0°). For the second repetition, we shift each row by 360/4 or 90° as described above for fig. 11.1. For the third and fourth repetitions we multiply each phase shift in the second repetition by 2 and 3 respectively. These four repetitions are diagrammatically represented in fig. 11.3 below. Note that in repetition 3, the difference between rows is 180°, and in repetition 4, it is 270°.

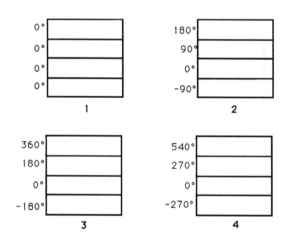

FIG. 11.3- PHASE SHIFTED ROWS FOR FOUR REPETITIONS
The shifts in repetition 3 are obtained by doubling the shifts in repetition 2; and the shifts in repetition 4 are obtained by tripling the shifts in repetition 2.

---

[*] This statement is an over-simplification for didactic purposes. It does not hold true for some of the techniques we will consider later.

Phase Encoding Repetitions and the Pixel Grid

If we go back to our 4 x 4 pixel grid, and if we consider the application of both the x gradient (frequency encoding) and the y gradient (phase encoding), then we can represent each pixel by a sine function of the appropriate frequency and phase shift. This is illustrated for each of the four phase encoding steps in figs. 11.4 to 11.7.

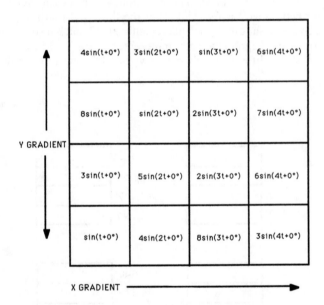

FIG. 11.4- FIRST REPETITION
The columns are frequency encoded but there is no phase shift of the rows.

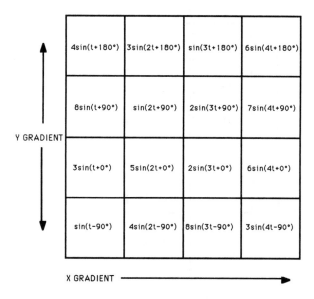

FIG. 11.5- SECOND REPETITION
The columns are frequency encoded and each row is phase shifted by 90° (360°/4).

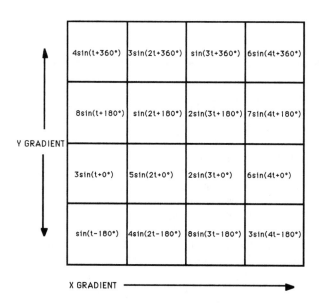

FIG. 11.6- THIRD REPETITION
The columns are frequency encoded and each row is phase shifted by 180° (twice the phase shift of the second repetition).

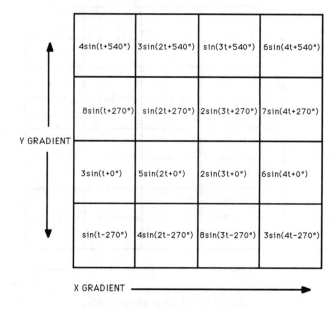

FIG. 11.7- FOURTH REPETITION
The columns are frequency encoded and each row is phase shifted by 270° (three times the phase shift of the second repetition).

Phase Encoding Repetitions and the MDM Vectors

Let us continue our hideously detailed coverage of frequency and phase encoding by showing what the precessing magnetic dipole moment vectors are doing in each of the 16 pixels in our example. We will let one vector represent all the vectors of a given pixel. We will consider two points in time, and we will show the position of the spinning vector at both these points in time: the position at the earlier point is represented by a solid arrow, and the position at the later point is represented by a broken arrow. This graphic device will replace the algebraic expression in each of the pixels in the figs. 11.4 thru 11.7. This is illustrated in figs. 11.8 thru 11.11 below.

Now let us look closely at figs. 11.8 thru 11.11. First, consider fig. 11.8. The solid arrow indicates the position of the MDM vector at the earlier point in time. Since this is the first repetition, there is no phase encoding, and therefore the solid arrow points in the same direction for all pixels. However, since there *is* frequency encoding along the x axis (horizontally), the vectors in each column are spinning at a different rate (from lesser to greater as one moves to the right). This is indicated by the fact that the angle between the initial (solid) arrow and later (broken) arrow increases for each column as we move from left to right. In other words, during a given time interval, the vector will have turned to a greater degree in those columns which are spinning at a faster rate. What we have done is to represent the precession frequency by showing the position of the MDM vector at two points in time.

Now if we consider figs. 11.9 thru 11.11, we see that the effect of phase encoding is to shift the position of the initial (and therefore of the later) vector. The amount of the shift differs between rows by 0° for the first repetition, 90° for the second, 180° for the third and 270° for the fourth. Note that even though the solid and broken arrows have been phase shifted, the angle between them is the same as in fig. 11.8, because the frequency encoding process does not vary from repetition to repetition.

It is necessary to point out that the order of phase encoding repetitions as presented here is not the order used by most commercial vendors. These scanners actually begin with the most positive (or negative) phase shifts and proceed through 0° to the opposite side. In our 4 x 4 pixel example, they would start with our 4th repetition and then continue with our first, second, and third.

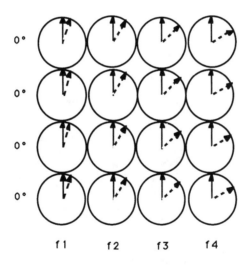

FIG. 11.8- FIRST REPETITION

There is no phase encoding, so the earlier vector position is at 12:00 for all rows. Note that the later vector position (broken arrow) becomes more advanced with each column to the right. This reflects the higher frequencies for those columns that are more to the right.

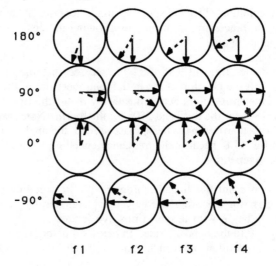

FIG. 11.9- SECOND REPETITION
This corresponds to fig. 11.5.

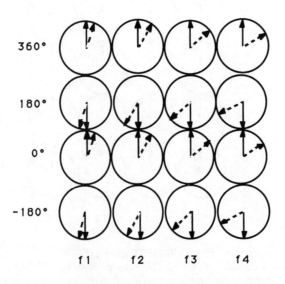

FIG. 11.10- THIRD REPETITION
This corresponds to fig. 11.6.

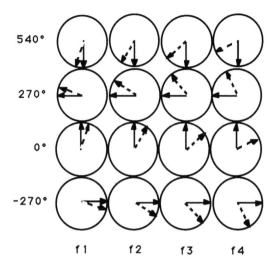

FIG. 11.11- FOURTH REPETITION
This corresponds to fig. 11.7.

Today's commercial MR scanners use many more phase encoding rows, i.e., repetitions, as well as frequency columns than in our 4 x 4 pixel grid example. Most scanners use 256 frequency gradations, and some multiple of 64 for the phase encoding rows (usually 128, 192 or 256)[*]. For example, if we are scanning with 256 phase encoding steps, then there will be 256 repetitions: the 128th repetition will have no phase shifts; the 129th will have each row shifted by 1.406° (360/256) with respect to its neighboring row; the 130th will have each row shifted by 2.812° (1.406 x 2) with respect to its neighbor; the 131st by 4.218° (1.406 x 3), etc.

In the next chapter, we will see how the signal is processed and how the 2DFT retrieves the image.

---

[*] Some vendors now allow any integral number of phase encoding steps up to 256.

12
Inside the "Black Box": From Signal to Image

We are now going to take a slightly different perspective by peering inside the scanner to see what it does from the time the raw signal is received to the final image. To some extent, we will be discussing the way the signals appear with some mathematical reference, but please do not become intimidated by this, for there is nothing here beyond simple high-school algebra. For some of you, this will be an important chapter, because it will bring to light some of the more mysterious terms you may have encountered in your reading- such as "real and imaginary signals" or "k-space", etc. And most important of all, we will examine the relationship of the 2DFT to the image.

Before we go any further, let us make sure we understand what a matrix is:

> In general, a matrix is a rectilinear array of elements. For our purposes, the only elements we will be considering will be numbers. Hence for us, a matrix is simply a set of numbers arranged in rows and columns.

Now the steps the scanner takes to achieve its goal of producing an image can be divided into three conceptual stages: (1) producing matrices where each row is a different repetition and each column is a point in time; (2) transforming these "repetition-time" matrices into matrices where each column is a frequency point and each row is a phase encoding angle; and (3) performing the 2DFT, which transforms these "phase-frequency" matrices into images, i.e., matrices whose rows and columns represent points on the x and y axis of the part being imaged. Each of these three steps will now be examined using the 4 x 4 pixel grid that formed the basis of our discussions up to now.

(1) **Repetition-Time Matrices**

Remember that with each pulse cycle, a phase encoding step is performed, and a signal is measured. That signal is a composite containing a "mini" signal contributed by each pixel. Now when the scanner "receives" a signal, what it is actually doing is recording the amplitude of the signal at equally spaced intervals in time. These interval measurements are known as "sampling points" or "samples" (fig. 12.1).[*]

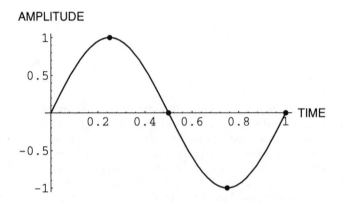

FIG. 12.1- SAMPLED POINTS ON A SINE CURVE
Four equally spaced points in time are sampled. If this were an MR signal, the row of data for this phase encoding step would be {1.0, 0, -1.0, 0}.

The scanner then stores its measurements as a matrix of data: each row of numbers represents a set of sampled points at equal intervals of time for each phase encoding step. In other words, each row is a different phase encoding step, and each column is a point in time in the measurement of the signals. It is this matrix of data that is known as "k-space".[**] It is important to realize that if we label the axes of this matrix, then the horizontal axis is time, and the vertical axis is repetition number. This matrix does not yet have any correspondence to spatial coordinates. Incidentally, this process of producing a data matrix from a received signal is *digitization.* This is an example of an analog to digital conversion.

---

[*] The number of sample points is usually twice the size of the matrix in the frequency direction, i.e., 512 samples for 256 frequency steps. We will say more about this later in the chapter on aliasing.

[**] The letter "k" comes from its use as a variable in the domain space of a Fourier transform.

Fig. 12.2 below shows graphs of the actual signal for our 4 x 4 pixel model for each phase encoding step. Each curve was obtained by simply plotting the sum of all the expressions for each of the figs. 11.4 through 11.7 respectively .

Each of the four signals shown in fig. 12.2 corresponds to each of the rows in the k-space matrix; so in a sense, the left side of fig. 12.2 shows a "graph" of k-space. Remember that although we visualize these signals as curves, the data in the scanner is simply a matrix of numbers.

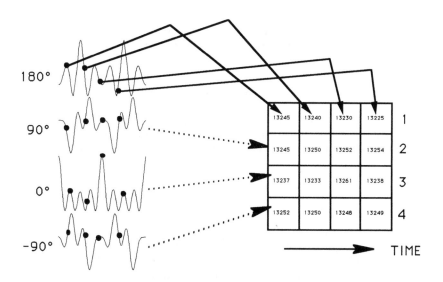

FIG. 12.2- RAW SIGNALS FOR THE 4 x 4 PIXEL GRID

Each curve is a graph of amplitude (y axis) vs. time (x axis) for each of the four phase encoding steps. The numbered degrees indicate the phase difference between rows for each phase shift (repetition). The data matrix is shown to the right. Its axes are repetition number vs. time. Its values come from the sampled points shown on the signal curves.

Splitting the Signal

Unlike a mathematical graph of a sine wave, there is no such thing as a starting point of a signal when it is received by the scanner. This means that the scanner has no idea whether or not the signal is phase shifted. For example, if we sample the curve sin(x) starting at one of its positive peaks, it will look identical to the curve sin(x+90°) with sampling starting at time 0 (fig. 12.3).

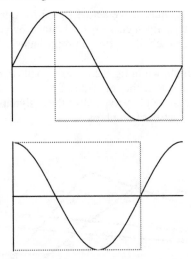

FIG. 12.3- SINE WAVES WITH 0° AND 90· PHASE SHIFTS
If each of the above signals is sampled within the gray square, the two data sets will be identical despite the fact that one signal is phase shifted 90° from the other.

In other words, the scanner needs to "ground itself" by relating the signal it is receiving to a known reference signal. This is done by subtracting a simple sine wave and a simple cosine wave from the received signal to obtain two separate signals from the original. In practice, a pure RF signal is used whose frequency is set to the Larmor frequency of hydrogen for the particular magnet being used, i.e., frequency of 64 MHz for a 1.5T magnet. Fig. 12.4 below shows the resultant rows of signals for our 4 x 4 pixel grid for each reference wave.

Note that it is customary to plot complex numbers with the real component on the x axis and the imaginary component on the y axis. Now since the cosine is maximum along the x axis, and the sine is maximum along the y axis, the signals resulting from subtraction of the cosine and sine waves have been termed "real" and "imaginary" signals respectively. However, there is nothing more real about one than the other; they might just as well have been called "x" and "y" or "sine" and "cosine" signals.

Note that once again, the bottom line for the scanner is a *matrix* of data whose vertical axis is repetition number and whose horizontal axis is time. However, we now have two matrices of data corresponding to the real and imaginary signals.

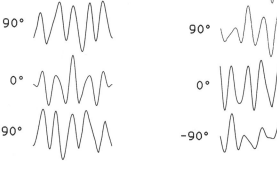
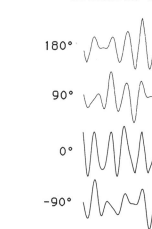

REAL   IMAGINARY

FIG. 12.4- REAL AND IMAGINARY "COMPONENTS" OF THE RAW SIGNAL
The functions cos(2.5x) and sin(2.5x) were each separately subtracted from the four
signals in fig. 12.2. The frequency of 2.5 was chosen because it represents the "center"
frequency of our pixel grid, whose frequencies range from 1 to 4. Note that in a real
scanner, 64 MHz for the reference RF signal should represent the "center" of the
frequency gradient (for a 1.5T magnet).

(2) Phase-Frequency Matrices

The First 1DFT

Almost immediately after the raw signal is split, a single dimensional Fourier
transform is obtained for both the "real" and "imaginary" components of the
signals. We demonstrated the application of a 1DFT (single dimensional Fourier
transform) in chapter 10, where we "transformed" a composite sine wave
function into spikes whose x coordinate represented the frequency and whose y
coordinate represented the amplitude for each of the component sine waves.
When this is done to the MR signal, we get a series of spikes corresponding to
the various frequencies of the signal for each phase encoding repetition for both
the real and imaginary signals. In our 4 x 4 model, this results in two blocks of 4
rows with 4 spikes per row[*] (fig. 12.5).

---

[*] Sort of. You may not see exactly 4 spikes because of inaccuracies of doing transforms
on a personal computer.

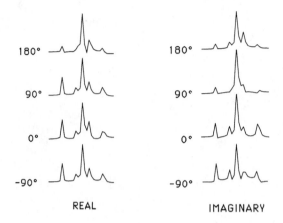

FIG. 12.5- 1DFT FOR THE REAL AND IMAGINARY SIGNALS FOR EACH OF
THE 4 PHASE ENCODING REPETITIONS

Note that what we mean when we say "do a transform on a row of data" is that
the numbers in that row are sequentially submitted to a computer algorithm to
produce a transform.

Once again, we emphasize that we are dealing with matrices of data. We now
have two matrices of "transformed" data: the vertical axes still represent
repetition number, but the horizontal axes now represent different frequencies
rather than points in time. The number entries represent the height of each spike
in the transform. We are half way towards producing a phase-frequency matrix,
i.e., we have a repetition-frequency matrix.

Combining the Data

This is a technical intermediate stage whereby the data in the two transformed
matrices from the last step are combined into one matrix. This is done by taking
the square root of the sum of the squares for each corresponding pixel in the two
matrices. This mathematical result is also known as the "modulus". When we
take the modulus of the two transformed matrices, we wind up with a third
matrix which is very similar to the two from which it came. Therefore, we are
still left with a "half-baked" repetition-frequency matrix.

The Second 1DFT

We must now take this matrix and transform each of the *columns* just the way
we transformed the rows in the first 1DFT. In other words, we will perform a
1DFT *perpendicular* to the way we did it earlier. That is, the numbers submitted

to the computer for each transform will come sequentially from each column of the matrix rather than from each row. This process will act upon the vertical axis, converting it from repetition number to phase encoding angle and hence yielding a "phase-frequency" matrix.

(3) Transformation to Image–The 2DFT

Why is the phase-frequency matrix so important? Because the phase frequency matrix is itself a two-dimensional Fourier transform; and in fact, it turns out to be the transform of the image matrix! To help understand why this is the case, remember that a Fourier transform is like a Fourier series (chapter 10); and a Fourier series is a sum of sines and cosines with increasing frequencies. And this is exactly what we get when we receive an MR signal. At the time of signal measurement, we apply a frequency or "read-out" gradient which imparts an increasing frequency to each column of spinning vectors, and our signal measurement is the sum of sines and/or cosines with multiple increasing frequencies. This is an over-simplification, since we are considering only the case of one dimensional transforms, but it is the same idea for the 2DFT.

Now remember that we stated earlier in chapter 10 that we can "toggle" back and forth between a function and its transform. That is, if F represents the transform of the function f, then the transform of F yields f, i.e., the transform of a transform of a function gives us back the original function. Therefore, since the phase-frequency matrix is a transform of the image, then if we take the transform of the phase-frequency matrix, we get back our image! Hence, we must apply a 2DFT to our phase-frequency matrix to convert it to a *spatial* matrix whose axes are the x and y spatial coordinates of the tissue we are seeking to image.

Now it is certainly beyond the scope of this book to mathematically show how a transform is done. However, we can come to an intuitive understanding of the relationship between the image and its 2DFT, the phase-frequency matrix. In chapter 10, we examined one dimensional transforms. Let us now give you an idea of what a 2DFT "looks like". Remember that a gray-scale image is a two-dimensional function. That is, for any specific values of two variables x and y, we get a third number, which is the value of the function. That function can be plotted in at least two ways: (1) as a surface in three dimensional space; and (2) as points of varying brightness on an x-y plane. The first type is called a "3D graph", and the second is known as a "density plot" or "gray-scale image". Nearly all images in radiology are density plots or gray-scale images; that is, they are three dimensional graphs utilizing two variables, which are plotted as points of varying brightness at each x,y location on a plane. Figs. 12.6 and 12.7 below plot the paraboloid function:

$$f(x,y) = 16 - x^2 - y^2$$

both as a surface in three dimensional space and as a density plot. The density plot version of this graph would be similar to a radiographic image of a paraboloid solid.

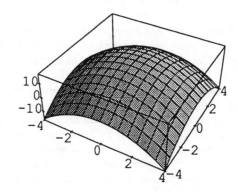

FIG. 12.6- PARABOLOID AS A GRAPH IN 3D SPACE

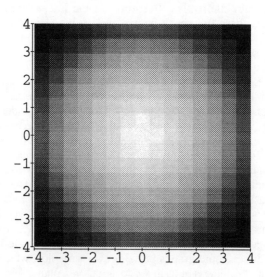

FIG. 12.7- PARABOLOID AS A DENSITY PLOT

Now a 2DFT of an image is also a two-dimensional function, and therefore it too can be graphed as either a surface or a density plot. Figs. 12.8 and 12.9 below show surface and density plot graphs respectively of a plane of finite area and its 2DFT.

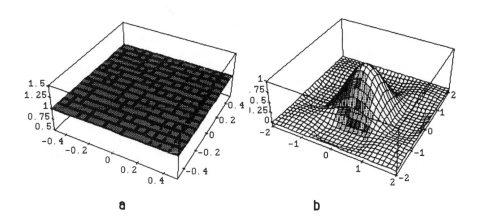

FIG. 12.8- 3D GRAPHS OF A PLANE AND ITS 2DFT

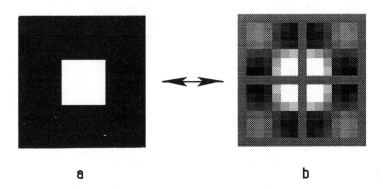

FIG. 12.9- DENSITY PLOTS OF A PLANE AND ITS 2DFT

The plane in "**a**" is the white square. It is considered as having a certain amplitude or height above some reference level, and therefore its image would be brighter than its surroundings.

The double arrow in fig. 12.9 illustrates the toggle nature of Fourier transforms: the square is the 2DFT of the figure labeled "b", and the figure labeled "b" is the 2DFT of the square. The phase-frequency matrix in the MR scanner bears the same relationship to the image matrix of the tissue being scanned as fig. 12.9b does to fig. 12.9a. Now we can see why we need a *two* dimensional Fourier transform to retrieve an image: because both the 2DFT and the radiographic image are functions of two variables.

At this point, we should say something more about k-space. Remember that k-space is the matrix of data that is initially obtained when the signal is measured: each element in the matrix is the amplitude of the signal at a point in time corresponding to the element's column, and for a repetition corresponding to the element's row. Now usually, the k-space matrix is obtained such that the columns on the left and the rows on the top are the most negative, the columns on the right and the rows on the bottom are the most positive, and zero lies somewhere at the center. When this is the case, it turns out that the centrally located rows and columns affect the contrast of the final image, whereas the peripheral rows and columns affect the detail or resolution of the image (fig. 12.10).

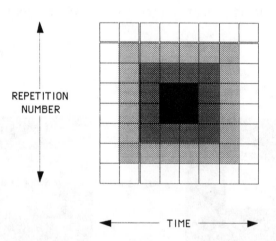

FIG. 12.10- k-SPACE MATRIX SHOWING REGIONS OF CONTRAST AND RESOLUTION

The darker the pixel, the more it affects contrast, and the lighter the pixel, the more it affects resolution.

In other words, k-space is essentially partitioned into regions which specialize in either contrast or resolution. We will see later that this theory is utilized in a breathing artifact suppression method as well as in a new, fast spin-echo technique.

Fig. 12.11 below summarizes the steps illustrated in this chapter.

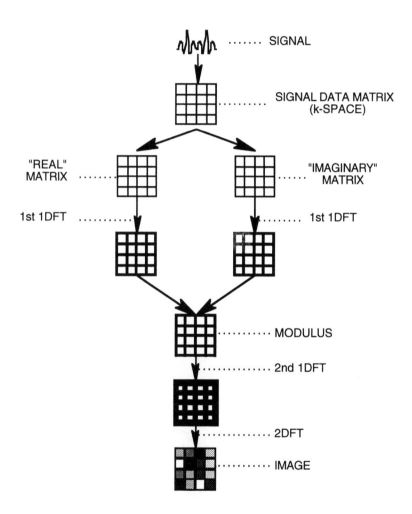

FIG. 12.11- SUMMARY OF SIGNAL PROCESSING STEPS
The thin line matrices have vertical and horizontal axes labeled "repetition number" and "time" respectively; the intermediate line matrices have axes labeled "repetition number" and "frequency"; and the heavy line matrix has axes labeled "phase" and "frequency".

13
Wrapping Up Basic Concepts

The Gradients in Perspective

We have seen that each of the three orthogonal gradients does a completely different job: the z gradient defines the slice; the x gradient imposes a frequency change; and the y gradient produces a phase change. It is important to realize that each gradient is the same physical phenomenon: a change in the magnetic field from one point in space to another. Also, each gradient produces the same basic effect on protons: the vector precession frequencies are changed. Therefore, the particular task each gradient performs is determined by essentially one thing: **when** in the pulse cycle the gradient is applied.

The z (slice select) gradient is applied only when the RF pulse is turned on; the x (frequency encoding) gradient is applied only when the signal is measured; and the y (phase encoding) gradient is applied briefly between the time the RF pulse is terminated and the signal is measured. How this causes each gradient to produce its effect has already been explained in previous chapters. Fig. 13.1a shows the temporal relationship of these three gradients to the other events in the spin-echo pulse cycle.

There is one other point of difference regarding the gradients. The frequency gradient and slice select gradient do not vary during an acquisition. On the other hand, the phase encoding gradient varies during the acquisition by increasing steadily with each phase shift repetition.

There is one other important relationship to be considered- between the steepness of the gradients and the field of view. Remember that once the slice select direction is determined, the frequency and phase encoding gradients frame out the image slice. Therefore, the field of view is directly related to the frequency and phase encoding gradients. And in fact, the smaller the field of view, the steeper the gradient. This is illustrated in fig. 13.1b below.

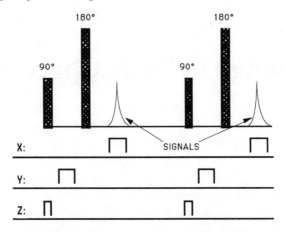

FIG. 13.1a- DOUBLE ECHO SPIN-ECHO PULSE CYCLE IN
RELATION TO GRADIENTS

The brackets indicate the x,y and z gradients. Note that the x gradient is applied only while the signals are received or read; the y gradient is applied after the RF pulses, but before the signals are measured; and the z gradient is applied only when the RF pulses are applied.

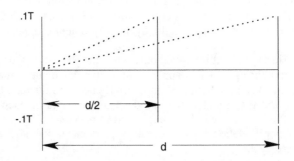

FIG. 13.1b- GRADIENT SLOPES FOR TWO FIELDS OF VIEW

The vertical axis is magnetic field strength in Tesla, and the horizontal axis is field of view size along one axis. The gradient slopes are indicated by the dotted lines. Note the steeper gradient for the smaller field of view.

If we consider all three gradients, then we see that the steeper the slice select gradient, the thinner the slice, and the steeper the frequency and phase encoding gradients, the smaller the field of view. Since steeper gradients require more power, this produces more strain on the gradients, and this explains why the practitioner occasionally encounters restrictions when attempting an image sequence with both thin slices and a small field of view.

Imaging in Other Planes

How do we produce images in the other orthogonal planes? The first thing to realize is that no matter what plane we image, the main external magnetic field always maintains its longitudinal orientation. This means, of course, that the z vectors are always "flipped" onto the x-y plane. What does change when we alter the plane of the image are the tasks we assign each **gradient** to perform. For example, if we wish to image in the coronal plane, then we will turn the y gradient on during the RF pulse to slice select; we could then apply the x gradient during the measurement of the signal to frequency encode; and apply the z gradient between the RF pulse and the signal measurement to phase encode. Note that we automatically establish the imaging plane by specifying which gradient is to be the slice select gradient. Once that is done, it makes no difference which of the other two remaining gradients is frequency or phase encoding. In our discussion of imaging in the axial plane, we could just as easily have assigned frequency to the y and phase to the x gradients. And in fact, commercial scanners allow the user the option to choose which way the frequency and phase encode axes will be oriented once the slice select axis is chosen.

What about oblique planes? Oblique planes are scanned by slice selecting in an oblique direction. By now, the reader may have been able to guess that this is done by applying two gradients **simultaneously** during the application of the RF pulse. Table 13.1 below summarizes how different planes are slice selected.

PLANE	IMAGE	SLICE SELECT GRADIENT
AXIAL		Z
CORONAL		Y
SAGITTAL		X
AXIAL OBLIQUE		Z + Y
CORONAL OBLIQUE		X + Y
SAGITTAL OBLIQUE		X + Z

TABLE 13.1–The column labeled "image" shows the orientation of the plane in question (dark line) with respect to two of the axes. The axes are defined as in chapter 3.

The Multislice Technique

Unlike CT scanning, the multiple slices of a spin-echo pulse sequence are not obtained one at a time. In other words, the scanner does not acquire all the information for a given slice before going on to the next slice. Remember that an image requires many repetitions of the RF pulses (as many as 256). Also, TR (time between repetitions) may be as long as 2000 ms for a T2 weighted study. That would require 2 x 256 = 512 seconds or 8.5 minutes to obtain that image. If we were to obtain 20 slices, then that sequence would take almost 3 hours, which would be prohibitively long.

Therefore, what the scanner does is the following. Since it has to wait 2 seconds before repeating the pulses on a given slice, it might as well acquire the first repetition for the other slices during that 2 second period of time. Then at 2 seconds (2000 ms), it will acquire the second repetition for the first slice. And again, since it must wait another 2000 ms, it will acquire the second repetition for the other slices, and so on. Hence, the scanner obtains a given repetition for **all** slices before going on to the next repetition. This is why the scanner is acquiring information on all the slices during the entire time the sequence is being obtained. This is illustrated in fig. 13.2 below.

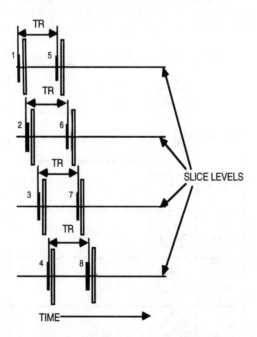

FIG. 13.2- MULTIPLE SLICES
There are four slices. Each pair of vertical skinny rectangles represents a 90°-180° spin-echo pulse cycle. The numbers represent the chronological sequence of the pairs of RF pulses. Note that the RF pulses occur at a slightly later time at each lower slice, but the TR intervals are equal for all slices.

A consequence of the above is that longer TR sequences will allow the scanner more time to acquire slices. We refer to this time as "sampling time". Hence, if we perform a T2 weighted sequence with a TR of 2000 ms, we will have a sampling time that is long enough to acquire as many as 20 slices; whereas, if we do a T1 weighted sequence with a TR of only 500 ms, we will not be able to obtain as many slices.

Note that the above discussion applies specifically to spin-echo pulse sequences. Many "fast scan" techniques utilize a TR as short as 20 ms. This does not allow enough sampling time to acquire other slices during that repetition time. Typically, these fast scan techniques acquire all the data on one slice before going on to the next–like the CT scanner.

Averages, Excitations

One more important miscellaneous concept to discuss regarding the MR scanner is that of "averages" or "number of excitations".[*] Basically, this refers to the number of times that the data is obtained or sampled. It is analogous to a researcher who makes several measurements of his data, and then averages them in order to obtain more precision. What the scanner does is to utilize multiple RF pulses and signal measurements **before** going on to the next phase encoding step.

For example, suppose that we are doing a single echo spin-echo with a 256 pixel matrix (i.e., there will be 256 rows in the phase encoding axis, and there will be 256 repetitions or "views"). Suppose, also, that we set the machine to do **two** excitations. Then, instead of just 256 pulse cycles (sets of 90°,180° pulses), there will be **512** pulse cycles–two for each of the 256 phase encoding steps. Hence the signal is measured 512 times–twice during each phase encoding step. These two signal measurements are then literally averaged, and this average result will be a statistical improvement over either of the two component measurements. If we had chosen **three** excitations, then of course there would be 768 pulse cycles –three for each of the 256 phase encoding steps.

Images obtained through the use of multiple excitations have a greater signal to noise ratio and usually appear "clearer" than those obtained with only one excitation. However, the time required for the acquisition becomes multiplied by the number of excitations chosen. Thus, a two excitation study takes twice as long as a one excitation exam, etc.

---

[*] Some manufacturers use the term "repetitions" to mean "excitations". This, of course, is confusing, since "repetition" is usually used to refer to the repeated pulse cycles, as we have described earlier.

Exam Time

The length of time for a given acquisition depends on just three user determined parameters: TR (time to repeat), number of phase encoding steps (or matrix size), and number of excitations. The product of these three yields the acquisition time:

$$\text{TIME IN MILLISECONDS} = TR * P * N$$

$$\text{TIME IN MINUTES} = TR * P * N \div 60000$$

where TR = time to repeat in milliseconds, P = number of phase encoding rows or steps (or repetitions), and N = number of excitations (or averages).

This is an important concept, for it means that no matter what equipment a scan was obtained on, if we know the TR, the matrix size (number of phase-encoding repetitions) and the number of excitations (signal averages), then we automatically know how long it took for that acquisition.

General Wrap-Up

That wraps it up for understanding the basic concepts of MR imaging in terms of the spin-echo pulse sequence. In Section III, we will address additional important MR topics, such as other pulse sequences and the effects of motion on the MR image. It is the author's contention that a thorough understanding of what has been presented up to now will provide the reader with a generic foundation that will enable him or her to deal effectively with the topics that are yet to be discussed.

SECTION III
Miscellaneous Topics

14
Some Other Pulse Cycles and Procedures

Inversion Recovery

The pulse cycle for inversion recovery consists of a 180° pulse followed by a 90° pulse (exactly the reverse of a spin-echo) followed by measurement of the signal. After the M vector is flipped 180°, it points directly downward in the z axis. As T1 relaxation occurs, the Mz vectors re-grow in a superior direction. After a period of time, the 90° pulse is applied and flips the partially reconstituted Mz vectors into the x-y plane. Since different tissues have different T1 relaxation times, the Mz vector for each tissue will be at a different height just before application of the 90° pulse, and therefore the resulting Mx vectors for the different tissues will have varying magnitudes reflecting the different T1's of the tissues. This is illustrated in fig. 14.1 below. Hence, the inversion recovery pulse sequence is one method of producing T1 weighted images. Often, the inversion recovery cycle described above is converted to a type of spin-echo by adding a 180° pulse. In that case, the pulse cycle would consist of a 180°, 90°, and then a sequence of 180° pulses.

In an inversion recovery pulse cycle, "TI" stands for "time to invert" and refers to the time between the 180° and 90° pulses. Note that in a T1 weighted image, substances with shorter T1's should have stronger signals. Hence we must have a long enough TI to allow the recovering Mz vectors to become positive (point upwards) before flipping them 90°. Later, we will consider a form of inversion recovery known as a "**STIR**" sequence, where a shorter TI is used as a method of suppressing fat.

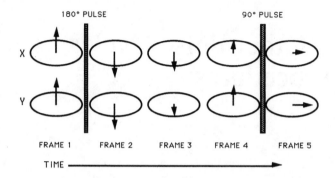

FIG. 14.1- SNAPSHOTS OF 2 TISSUES DURING INVERSION RECOVERY
Note that Y's Mz vector recovers faster than X's and therefore has a shorter T1. If we wait long enough for both Mz vectors to become positive (frame 4), then Y's Mz vector will be taller than X's, and when they are flipped, Y's signal will be stronger. If we applied our 90° pulse between frames 3 and 4, then the substance with the longer T1 would have a stronger signal, and this would not yield a T1 weighted image. Hence we must have a relatively long TI to produce a T1 weighted image.

Fast Scans

This pulse cycle is more commonly used, but is more difficult to completely understand. This is the so called "fast scan" or "gradient field echo". Two common acronyms are "GRASS"™ (General Electric, Milwaukee) and "FLASH", which stand for **G**radient **R**ecalled **A**cquisition at **S**teady **S**tate and **F**ast **L**ow **A**ngle **SH**ot, respectively.

Now the whole idea behind fast scanning is to make the scan fast. And this is done essentially by using an ultra-short TR. But in order to do this, two things must be done. First of all, the flip angle must be less than 90°. If we were to use a 90° flip angle with a very short TR, we would not allow the Mz component of the M vector to recover sufficiently between pulse cycles to yield an adequate signal; but if we use a *reduced* flip angle, then the Mz component of the M vector is not decreased very much by the flip (fig. 14.2).

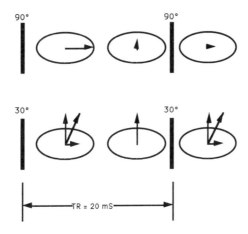

FIG. 14.2- PARTIAL FLIP vs. 90° FLIP

With the 90° flip, the entire M vector is flipped horizontal leaving no vertical component; and if the TR is short (20 mS), then re-growth of the vertical component must be limited, and subsequent 90° flips will yield a small signal. But with the 30° flip, a significant vertical component remains, and subsequent flips would therefore yield a larger signal.

Secondly, if we study fig. 14.2, we realize that when the vector is flipped less than 90°, we are left with both a horizontal and a vertical component of the flipped M vector. If we were to then apply a 180° refocusing pulse, it would flip *both* of those vectors 180°, resulting in two right angle vectors, and this would interfere with obtaining a proper signal. Therefore, we must eliminate the 180° refocusing pulse if we are to use less than 90° flip angles; and we must use less than 90° flip angles if we wish to significantly shorten our TR and hence our scan time.

In order to measure the non-re-focused FID signal, fast scans make use of a modified frequency gradient: one that consists of a negative gradient followed by a positive gradient of equal strength, but applied twice as long. Remember from chapter 9 that when the frequency gradient is applied, each column of MDM vectors perpendicular to the direction of the gradient will be spinning at a different frequency. Consider the effect of the fast scan gradient on one of these columns whose frequency we will call f (fig. 14.3).

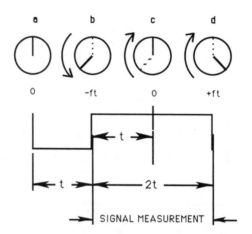

FIG. 14.3- FAST SCAN GRADIENT REFOCUSING

At **a**, there is no phase shift (vector at 12:00). At **b**, after time t, the negative gradient has caused a phase shift of -120° (vector has moved counter-clockwise to 8:00). Now the positive gradient is applied, equal in strength to the negative. This causes the spins to immediately reverse their direction, while spinning at the same frequency. Therefore at **c**, after another time t, the phase is shifted +120° back to its starting point (vector has moved clockwise to 12:00), and this is in the center of the time span of the signal measurement. This is the principle of gradient refocusing. At **d**, the end of the signal measurement, the vector is phase shifted to +120°. Note the symmetry: at the beginning of signal measurement, the phase is -120°, and at the end it is +120°; but in the middle, there is no phase shift.

First the negative gradient is applied for a time t. According to our concept of phase as frequency times time, we get a phase shift of -ft. Next we apply a positive gradient of the same strength. During this positive component of the gradient, we measure the signal. *Half* way through the application of this positive gradient, another time period of t will have passed. The new phase shift will therefore be +ft. This will exactly cancel out the -ft phase shift for the negative gradient, and hence there will be no phase shift at the mid-point of the time we are reading the signal. This argument applies to each frequency of each column along the frequency axis. This is the principal of the "gradient echo":

The bi-lobed fast scan frequency gradient causes all spins to be in phase at the center of the time span for the measurement of the signal.

Note that we are not really **re-focusing** the spins, for that would require a 180° pulse. The fast scan gradient is simply a technique that allows measurement of the FID signal in the absence of a 180° re-focusing pulse.

Fig. 14.4 shows a schematic representation of a fast scan pulse cycle.

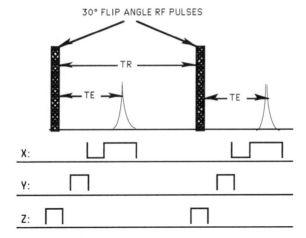

FIG. 14.4- DIAGRAM OF FAST SCAN PULSE CYCLE WITH 30° FLIP
The gradients are indicated by brackets. Note that the frequency (x axis) gradient is "bi-lobed". It consists of a negative gradient for time t (open bracket at top) followed by an equal magnitude positive gradient for time 2t (open bracket at bottom) centered around the time the signal is to be measured. Note that there is no 180° refocusing pulse, but we have a TR and a TE, just like a spin-echo.

Now, because there is no 180° refocusing pulse, the signal intensity that is measured for a given substance (such as water) cannot be thought of as representing a point on a true T2 curve. The signal intensity that is measured is simply that of T2*–the signal that results from free induction decay. Therefore, we encounter a problem if we attempt to apply the concept of T2 weighting to a fast scan image.   Now we *can* assess the degree of T2* weighting on a fast scan, and this is analogous to how we did it for T2 weighting: the longer the TR, and the TE, the greater the T2* weighting. To the extent to which T2* curves of different substances correlate with their respective T2 curves, we can expect the image contrast to behave similarly to a spin-echo sequence as TE is manipulated. However, we certainly cannot rely on this, and therefore, we should really speak of *T2** weighting and not T2 weighting when analyzing fast scan images.

It is important to realize that T2* decay is much more rapid than T2 decay, and therefore, we cannot use the relatively long TE values that we used with spin-echo imaging, or else our images would have so little signal that they would look too noisy or grainy to read. Hence most fast scans are performed with TE's of approximately 10-15 milliseconds, rather than values of 20-80 milliseconds, which are typically used with spin-echo pulse sequences.

The situation for T1 weighting in fast scans is different from that of T2 weighting. Re-polarization of the Mz vector occurs during the TR period of a fast scan just as it does in a spin-echo sequence. Therefore, the concept of T1 weighting does apply to fast scan imaging: the shorter the TR, the greater the T1 weighting.

Also, shorter flip angles tend to result in less T1 weighting. This is because with shorter flip angles, the resultant vertical Mz vector remains large. It therefore has less to recover before the next pulse cycle. Therefore, tissues with longer T1 relaxation times will have Mz vectors that recover to the same extent as tissues with shorter T1 relaxation times. Hence tissues with different T1 relaxation rates will not be differentiated, and therefore there will be less T1 weighting.

Fig. 14.5 shows graphs of relative signal intensity vs. flip angle in a fast scan for water, fat and muscle.

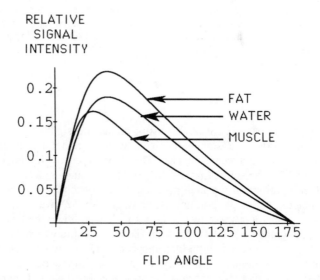

FIG. 14.5- SIGNAL INTENSITY CURVES vs. FLIP ANGLE FOR TR=30ms

These curves were generated using TR = 30ms without considering the T2* values for the different substances. We can think of the graphs as representing signal intensities obtained with negligible or very small TE's (remember that with a small TE, we do not allow much time for T2* decay, and therefore T2* would have a negligible influence on the relative signal intensities). Note that there is a maximum of signal intensity and contrast with flip angles around 40-

60°. The reader should beware that for most typical fast scan sequences, the signal intensities of water and fat on the resulting images will not match the curves in the above figure: water will have a higher intensity than other substances. This is because we are showing signal intensity curves independent of T2*, and a typical fast scan with a TE of 15ms will allow the T2* effects of the different tissues to influence the image contrast.

Fast scans are just that—fast. This is because there is no 180° re-focusing pulse, and the TR can be extremely short, perhaps as low as 20 ms (1/100 the TR for a T2 weighted spin-echo). Most spin-echo acquisitions take upwards of 3-4 minutes. However, a fast scan with only a 20-30° flip angle and a TR of 20 ms may yield 15-20 slices in only 30 seconds. So fast scans may be useful for abdominal examinations, since the patient would be able to hold his breath for the entire acquisition.

It is of interest that fast scan *slices* are acquired differently from spin-echo sequences. Remember that for spin-echo pulse sequences, the so-called "multi-slice" technique is used, whereby multiple slices are excited during a given TR interval (pulse cycle), which means that data is being acquired for each slice during the entire acquisition. However, with fast scans, all of the data for each slice is acquired before proceeding to the next slice. This is probably a consequence of the fact that there would be little time to excite other slices during the ultra-short TR's that are typical of fast scanning. Note that because of this concept, we can shorten a fast scan sequence by simply decreasing the number of slices; whereas decreasing the number of slices has no effect on the exam time of a typical multi-slice spin-echo sequence.

There is one more very important property of fast scans: they tend to produce an intense signal in vascular structures. This will be considered later, when we discuss the appearance of moving blood on the MR image.

Summary of Fast Scan Ideas

(1) Fast scans are fast.
(2) Flip angles of approximately 40-60° produce the greatest overall signal strength.
(3) The greater the TR, the less the T1 weighting, as with the spin-echo.
(4) Shorter flip angles result in less T1 weighting.
(5) The concept of T2 weighting should be replaced by the concept of T2* weighting when analyzing fast scans.
(6) Fast scans tend to produce intense signals in arteries and veins.
(7) Fast scans are acquired one slice at a time.

Pulse Cycle Summary

The following is a summary of all the pulse cycles that we have so far described:

Spin-echo: {90°, 180°, (180°), (180°), ...}

Inversion Recovery: {180°, 90°, (180°), (180°),...}

Fast Scan: {<90°}

Three Dimensional Fourier Imaging

Up to now, our concept of imaging involved the use of a gradient to select the slices and the application of frequency and phase encoding to map the spatial information on each slice. This necessitated the use of a two dimensional Fourier transform (2DFT) to decode this information into a recognizable image for each slice. With a procedure known as *three* dimensional Fourier transform (3DFT) imaging, the slice-select gradient is no longer employed for each individual slice. Instead, a single slice is selected that is thick enough to contain the first and last slices of the desired imaging volume; and then each of the three orthogonal axes is encoded: frequency along the x axis and phase along the y *and the z axis*. Now since all **three** orthogonal axes are encoded (not just x and y), a **three** dimensional Fourier transform is necessary to decode this information.

Here is how this works in greater detail. Recall that the slice select gradient is imposed along the z axis at the time of the 90° RF pulse, and the thickness of the slices is determined by the steepness of the gradient: the steeper the gradient, the thinner the slice. In a 3DFT sequence, a very shallow slice-select gradient is applied so that a relatively thick slice is selected along the z axis (as thick as the volume of tissue to be sliced). Remember also that in a 2DFT sequence, the phase encoding gradient is applied between the 90° and 180° RF pulses. Now in a *3DFT* sequence, *both* the y axis and the z axis gradients are both applied sometime between the 90° and 180° RF pulses. For the same reasons that the y axis becomes phase encoded, so does the z axis. Fig. 14.6 shows a summary of this process.

The number of phase encoding steps for the z axis is specified by the user. However, it does not necessarily determine the number of *slices*. The 3DFT process yields a *volume* of tissue, which is subsequently sliced mathematically by the user for as many slices and in any direction that he (or she) wishes. The number of phase encoding steps in the z axis will ultimately play a role in determining the resolution in the z axis as a function of the slice thickness. Hence, if the number of z axis phase encoding steps is less than the number of z axis slices subsequently chosen by the user, then the resultant images may not accurately reflect the desired slice thickness.

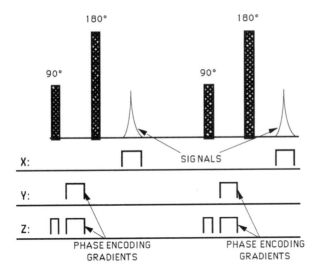

FIG. 14.6- TWO 3DFT PULSE CYCLES

The skinny z gradient preceding the phase encoding gradient is used to select the single slice for the volume to be imaged. It is, of course, applied during the 90° RF pulse. The x gradient is the read-out gradient, just as for a 2DFT pulse cycle.

The exam time for a 3DFT imaging sequence is calculated in an analogous fashion to that for the spin-echo sequence, except for the additional factor for the number of z axis encoding steps. You can think of it as consisting of a 2DFT sequence time for *each* phase encoding step in the z axis. Therefore, the exam time is equal to the exam time for a 2DFT sequence times the number of phase encoding steps in the z direction:

$$\text{TIME IN MINUTES} = TR * Py * Pz * N \div 60000$$

where TR is the repetition time in milliseconds, Py is the number of phase encoding steps in the y axis, Pz is the number of phase encoding steps in the z axis, and N is the number of excitations or signal averages.

The main advantage of this procedure is that once the imaging volume is obtained, any number of sets of very thin contiguous slices in any direction may then be produced without additional pulse sequences. The disadvantage is that it can take a long time to obtain the imaging volume. For example, a standard 2DFT spin-echo sequence with a matrix size of 256, 1 signal average and a TR = 2000 will yield about 18 slices in approximately 8 1/2 minutes. However, if we obtain the same T2 weighted sequence using 18 phase encoding increments in the z axis, the total time is nearly 3 *hours*. Therefore, it is impractical to use a standard spin-echo sequence with 3DFT imaging, and fast scan techniques are usually employed. Also, we will see later that 3DFT sequences can be used for MR angiography.

Half Fourier Imaging

So called "half Fourier transform" imaging is a process that reduces scanning time. Suppose that it takes 4 minutes using a certain TR to create a scan with a matrix size of 40 with one signal average.* Suppose also that we wish to cut the imaging time in half. Now of course, we could either halve the TR or halve the number of phase encoding steps to accomplish that end. However, if we reduce TR, we will reduce the degree of T2 weighting, and if we reduce the number of phase encoding steps, we will reduce our matrix size and decrease the resolution (this concept to be discussed later). Half Fourier transform imaging allows us to cut the scanning time in half without altering either the TR or the matrix size. Here is how it works.

Recall that phase encoding is performed over a 360° cycle. This means that for a matrix of 40, there will be 40 phase encoding steps of 9° each. Also, remember that this is accomplished by going from -180° through 0° to +171° (chapter 11). With half Fourier transform imaging, only half of that cycle is performed, and the other half is extrapolated mathematically. For example, the phase encoding would be applied from 0° to 171° in steps of 9°, for a total of 20 steps. Then the data for the steps from -9° to -180° are determined from this information (c.f. fig. 14.7).

Referring to fig. 14.7, it turns out that the data in the "lower" half of the matrix is related to the data in the "upper" half by a kind of symmetrical relationship. In fact, the data in the pixels of the lower half of the matrix tend to be the same as the data in the upper half; it is simply arranged in a different rectilinear pattern. For a given pixel in the upper half with coordinates x and y, there will be a pixel in the lower half with the same signal intensity value, except that it will be located at -x,-y. This is illustrated by the small black boxes in fig. 14.7. It turns out that the position of the two black boxes illustrates the relationship of radial symmetry: if we draw lines connecting each box with the origin, the two lines are equal in length and exactly 180° apart. Incidentally, note that the lines of data in fig, 14.7 are what is known as "k-space", as we described in chapter 12. What we are saying is that k-space is theoretically a radially symmetric matrix of data.

In this process, we see that only 20 rather than 40 phase encoding steps are performed, and hence the sequence takes only half as long to acquire. Note that although we do not disturb the TR and matrix size, the resulting image does have a lower signal-to-noise ratio than the original 2DFT sequence. In fact, the

---

* This matrix size is unrealistic. However, it was chosen so that the accompanying illustration would be able to show all the phase encoding steps.

signal-to-noise ratio is decreased in the same proportion as if we had cut our signal averages from 4 to 2, or from 2 to 1, etc. Hence it is as if we did cut our averages from 1 to 1/2; and indeed, some refer to half Fourier imaging as "half-NEX" imaging (where "NEX" refers to "Number of EXcitations").

It is important to realize that in half-Fourier transform imaging, the matrix size is twice the number of repetitions, and therefore the two are not equal. Therefore, we must modify the formulas for acquisition time given in chapter 13 by including an additional factor of 0.5.

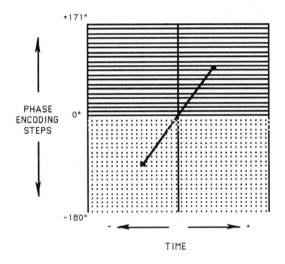

FIG. 14.7- HALF FOURIER IMAGING
This is a diagram of k-space. The phase encoding steps are along the vertical axis from -180° to +171°. The solid horizontal lines in the upper half of the matrix represent the data along the time axis for the phase encoding steps that are actually performed, and the dotted horizontal lines in the lower half represent the extrapolated data. The tiny square in the right upper quadrant of the matrix represents an actual data measurement; the tiny square in the left lower quadrant represents the same data value, but transposed to a different location according to radial symmetry (c.f. text).

Echo Planar Imaging

Echo planar or "fast spin-echo" imaging is a technique for producing standard appearing spin-echo images with a dramatic reduction in imaging time. The way it works is as follows. Consider the case of a standard quadruple spin-echo technique with TE's of 20, 40, 60 and 80 ms. Recall that for each phase encoding step, we measure the MR signal at each of these TE time intervals, so that all four of the signal intensity measurements are obtained with the same phase encoding step. The final image requires a certain number of these phase encoding steps–say 256, for example. Now suppose that we change the phase encoding gradient for each of the four TE time steps (fig. 14.8).

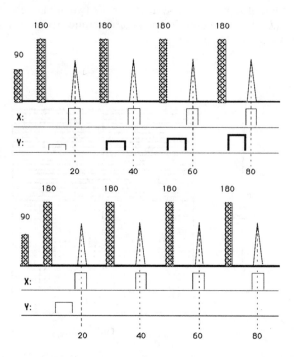

FIG. 14.8- DIAGRAMS OF CONVENTIONAL AND FAST SPIN-ECHO
The higher diagram is a fast spin-echo. Note that the Y phase encoding gradient is applied (and *increased*) after each 180° pulse in the pulse cycle. The lower diagram is a conventional spin-echo, where the Y gradient is applied only once in the pulse cycle.

We have now acquired the same imaging information as we would have in the first four phase encoding steps of a conventional spin-echo sequence; but we have done it in the time that it takes for only one of those steps. In other words, if our TR is 2000 ms, then it would take four repetitions (eight seconds) to acquire 4 phase encoding steps in the conventional spin-echo as opposed to only one repetition (two seconds) with echo planar imaging. Hence we would cut our imaging time to 1/4 the time for the standard spin-echo sequence. Of course, there is nothing special about the number 4; we could use any number of signal measurements and phase encoding steps, as long as there is enough time within the pulse cycle[*] to fit them in.

Several things need to be pointed out at this juncture. First of all echo planar images are true spin-echo images, in which a 180° pulse precedes each signal measurement (unlike "fast scan" or gradient echo images). Also, there is no sacrifice of statistical information as there is, for example, with half Fourier imaging (p. 112). We get all the information of a conventional spin-echo. However, nature does not usually give us something for nothing: with echo planar imaging, we only get one image per slice location- as opposed to four in the case of a conventional quadruple multi-echo.

Second, we must realize that echo planar images are composed of a "hybrid" of TE signal samples. In other words, in a conventional spin-echo sequence, a given image is created from signal intensity measurements all obtained at the same TE, whereas in echo planar imaging, the information constituting the image comes from signals measured at different TE's. Now it is possible to create an image with the characteristics of a given TE by re-ordering the phase encoding steps such that the more central phase encoding steps correspond in time to the TE in question. This principle is similar to that used in respiratory ordered phase encoding (p. 139). This is an example of utilizing the theory that k-space can be partitioned into regions that "specialize" in contrast or resolution (p. 92).

---

[*] Remember that a pulse cycle is a repeating unit of radiofrequency pulse and signal measurements (p. 33).

15
Matrix Size and the Field of View

In this chapter, we will examine the effect of matrix size and field of view on the quality of the image. Many of the basic ideas here are applicable to other imaging modalities, such as CT scanning.

The Pixel

Let us begin by thinking of the pixel, as discussed in chapter 9, as the fundamental unit or building block of the image. The image cannot be broken down into any elements smaller than the pixel. This means that the image characteristics cannot vary *within* a pixel, for the pixel is all one density: either black or white in a monochrome image, a particular shade of gray in a gray scale image such as a radiograph or MRI image, or a particular color in a color image.

There are two image quality concepts that we will relate to the size of the pixel: resolution and noise.

Resolution

We want the notion of resolution to somehow be a measure of the detail of an image. This is usually done by defining resolution to be the minimum distance that two lines can be perceived or distinguished. The smaller that distance is, the greater the resolution. Now since image characteristics cannot vary within a pixel, the size of the pixel will determine how much detail or resolution the image can have: if the interval between two lines is smaller than the size of two adjacent pixels, the lines will not be perceived as separate (fig. 15.1). We therefore come to an important conclusion regarding MR scanning (and other modalities as well):

> The smaller the pixel, the greater the resolution of the image.

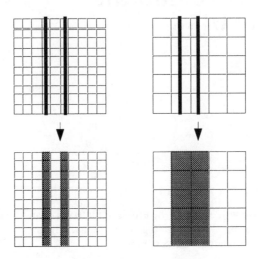

FIG. 15.1- RESOLUTION AND PIXEL SIZE
On the left, the pixels are small enough to allow a column between the 2 lines, and hence the lines can be resolved. On the right, the pixels are too large, and the 2 lines appear as one fat line.

Noise

Consider a slab or block to be imaged. That block will generate a certain amount of signal intensity which will be represented by a rectangular region of the image. Now let us think of this signal intensity as composed of many tiny packets of energy which will be distributed to all the pixels in the rectangular image of the block. Without getting into the mathematics of statistics, we all know that for a given study or experiment, the smaller the sample, the less valid are the results. Therefore, if the pixels are small, then there will be fewer energy packets distributed to each pixel, simulating the situation of a study or experiment with few samples. Hence the "value" or density assigned to each pixel is less reliable. This causes a variation in density from one pixel to the next, which in turn yields a grainy effect, which is referred to as "noise" or "quantum mottle".

Now let us consider the hypothetical situation of two adjacent blocks, each 10 mm in thickness, such that one block has twice the signal intensity of the other (fig. 15.2). We will suppose for argument's sake that the left block has a signal intensity of 64 (arbitrary) units, and the right block has a signal intensity of 32 units. Now we divide each block into a grid of 4 pixels (situation 1). When a 10 mm thick MR image is produced, the total amount of the signal intensity for each block will be essentially distributed among the pixels resulting in 16 units/pixel (64/4) for the left block and 8 units/pixel (32/4) for the right block.

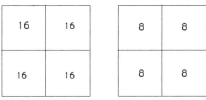

SITUATION 1

4	4	4	4
4	4	4	4
4	4	4	4
4	4	4	4

2	2	2	2
2	2	2	2
2	2	2	2
2	2	2	2

SITUATION 2

FIG. 15.2- VARYING THE MATRIX SIZE FOR TWO CONTRASTING BLOCKS
In each situation, the left sided block has twice the signal intensity of the right block. However, the *difference* in density between the two blocks is greater for the larger pixel size (situation 1) than for the smaller (situation 2). Hence statistical variation may make it more difficult to distinguish the two blocks in situation 2 than in situation 1.

However, if, we divide each block into 16 pixels (situation 2), each pixel in the left block will have 4 units (64/16), and each pixel in the right block will have 2 units (32/16). We see that the difference in signal intensity (4 minus 2) between the blocks in situation 2 is less than it is in situation 1 (16 minus 8). Now since the pixels are smaller in situation 2 than in situation 1, there will be more noise or statistical variation in the density of the pixels in situation 2. Furthermore, since the difference in signal intensity between the two blocks is less in situation 2, the statistical variation that does occur among the pixels will tend to even out the signal intensity difference between the pixels in the two blocks. This will decrease contrast. This leads us to another conclusion:

The smaller the pixel, the greater the noise and the less the contrast of the image.

Note that were it not for the statistical variation described above, the contrast between the two blocks would be the same for the two situations: 16/8 = 4/2.

Varying the Pixel Size

There are basically two ways of doing this: changing the matrix size or changing the field of view. Think of the situation as analogous to tiling a room: the pixels are the tiles, and the field of view is the room size. So if we increase the matrix size while holding the field of view constant, we decrease the pixel size (tiling the same size room with more tiles: the tiles have to be smaller); and if we decrease the field of view while holding the matrix size constant, we decrease the pixel size (the tiles have to be smaller in order for the same number to fit a smaller room–fig. 15.3).

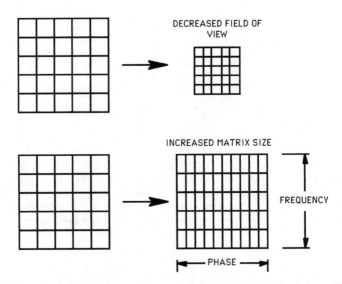

FIG. 15.3- FIELD OF VIEW vs. MATRIX SIZE
If we decrease the field of view while holding the matrix size constant (top situation) or if we increase the matrix size while holding the field of view constant (bottom situation), we decrease the pixel size (although in the second case, the decrease occurs only in the horizontal axis, because matrix size is usually increased by changing only the number of phase encoding steps).

Note that there are several important conceptual differences between altering the field of view and altering the matrix size: (1) changing the matrix size alters the time of the examination but not the area being examined; (2) changing the field of view alters the anatomical area being imaged but does not change the time; (3) changing the matrix size changes the pixel size only in the phase encoding direction, whereas changing the field of view changes the pixel size in both directions. However, whether this results in a perceptual difference is questionable. Note that since the size of the matrix in the frequency direction is usually a constant 256, the only MR images with square pixels are those in which the phase encoding matrix size is set at 256 (usually 256 repetitions).

Large vs. Small Pixel Images

In our routine scanning, we sometimes obtain a suboptimal image as a function of an inappropriate pixel size. It is crucial to be able to recognize from the image whether the pixel is too big or too small so that the appropriate pixel size alteration can be made (by changing the field of view and/or the matrix size).

If the pixel size is too large, the image will lack resolution and will appear blurry or as if it were out of focus. You might think that the larger pixel size would cause the image to look jagged as a result of visualizing the individual enlarged pixels. However, this is usually not the case because of the high resolution of the viewing monitors and techniques which serve to "smooth" the image so that the pixels are not seen. The net result is an image that lacks resolution, which is perceived as a sort of out of focus picture.

If the pixel size is too small, then the image will appear grainy or speckly rather than out of focus.

The author has created a computer program that randomly distributes "energy packets" to a pixel grid. In fig. 15.4, the program was used to distribute 200 particles to a rectilinear area with a matrix size of 10 x 10.[*] If a particle hit a certain square region within the area, it was assigned a higher value, thereby simulating a region of higher signal intensity.

---

[*] The gray scale graphs were created using *Mathematica* ™, Wolfram Research, Inc., Champaign, IL.

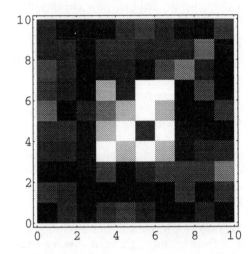

FIG. 15.4- 200 PARTICLES, 10 x 10 MATRIX
Note the central square of higher signal intensity is fairly easy to perceive.

In fig. 15.5 below, the same experiment was performed using a 20 x 20 matrix.

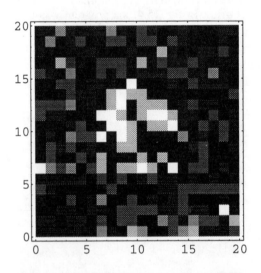

FIG. 15.5- 200 PARTICLES, 20 x 20 MATRIX
Note that the statistical variation caused by the smaller pixel size renders the central high signal intensity square less well visualized.

Notice how difficult it is to see the central square on the 20 x 20 matrix, because of the statistical variation of the smaller pixels. We have essentially simulated a grainy appearance.

Now as an aside, remember that we can improve our statistics by using more samples. In fig. 15.6, we used 800 particles, which lessens the statistical variation and renders the central square more apparent.

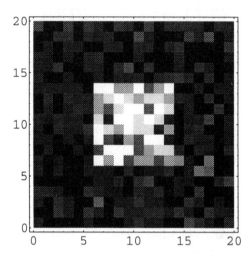

FIG. 15.6- 800 PARTICLES, 20 x 20 MATRIX

In an MR scan, we can do the same sort of thing by increasing our number of signal averages. Also, remember from chapter 6 that increasing TR or decreasing TE increases signal intensity, and this is just like having a greater number of energy packets to distribute, which would reduce mottle or noise. (Of course, contrast would be modified by other factors related to relaxation times.) Finally, thicker slices result in an overall greater signal intensity, which tends to reduce quantum mottle.

Rectangular Field of View

Normally, if we try to reduce the time of an MRI sequence by decreasing the number of phase encoding steps, we will also reduce the matrix size, increase the pixel size, and consequently decrease resolution, which we may not wish to do. Now it is true that we can decrease our field of view as well as our matrix size, thereby preserving the pixel size and yet decreasing the number of phase encoding steps and therefore the time of the examination sequence. However, this may give us a field of view that is simply too small for our needs. With rectangular field of view, we halve the field of view only in the phase encoding direction, and halve the number of phase encoding steps (fig. 15.7). This preserves the pixel size while cutting the time of the sequence in two. The resulting image is a rectangle that is half the area of the original square field of view. The size in the frequency direction is not altered.

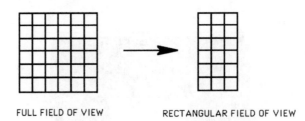

FULL FIELD OF VIEW   RECTANGULAR FIELD OF VIEW

FIG. 15.7- RECTANGULAR FIELD OF VIEW
The rectangular field of view is half the size and contains half the number of pixels. Hence the pixel size is unchanged.

This technique is particularly suitable for sagittal images of the spine, where a rectangular field would easily accommodate the shape of the area of interest. If we did not have access to rectangular field of view, and if we chose to halve the field of view (and decrease our matrix size), we would cut *both* axes of our view in two and wind up with a square field of view 1/4 the area of the original. This would probably not be appropriate for a sagittal spine image.

Summary

The following is a tabular summary of the above described parameters with respect to resolution and noise ("↑" means increased, "↓" means decreased, and "0" means unchanged):

	RESOLUTION	NOISE
↑ MATRIX SIZE	↑	↑
↑ FIELD OF VIEW	↓	↓
↑ NSA	0	↓
↑ TR	0	↓
↑ TE	0	↑
↑ SLICE THICKNESS	0	↓

16
Motion

General Considerations

In this chapter, we will discuss the very important topic of how moving entities affect the MR image. We will cover general principles, flowing blood, and devices used to control motion artifacts. MR angiography will be treated in the next chapter. Although we will try to explain every phenomenon in terms of the principles that we have already learned, this may not always be possible because of the complexity of this subject. However, we will be able to explain most things; and we will be sure to acknowledge those instances where we fall short of an adequate explanation.

Two Types of Motion Artifact

To begin with, motion nearly always produces some form of artifact on the MR image. Now when we say "artifact", we refer to the appearance of something on the image which does not represent or correlate with anything real in the volume of tissue being imaged. Whenever anything moves during a spin-echo pulse sequence, two basic types of motion artifact are produced: (1) a blurring of the moving object **in the direction that the object is moving,** and (2) a blurring or image of the moving object **along the phase encoding direction,** no matter which way the object is moving.

The first type of motion artifact is relatively easy to understand and is analogous to the blurred image we would get if we photographed a rapidly moving object using a relatively slow shutter speed. In other words, as the object moves while we try to image it, we sort of "catch" it in different locations, creating a blurring effect.

The second type of artifact is more difficult to comprehend. Once again, we must return to our familiar Larmor equation: the frequency of precession of the MDM vectors is directly proportional to the strength of the magnetic field. Now during any MR sequence we are constantly applying magnetic field gradients in all three orthogonal directions. Therefore, if something moves along the axis of one of the applied gradients, it will experience a variation in the magnetic field, and hence its MDM vectors will likewise experience a variation in their spin frequency. This will alter the phase of the MDM vectors in this moving object. Now since, as we saw earlier, we use phase to "label" positions in the phase encoding direction, the moving object will be mislabeled in that direction (because its phase has been altered), and we will get artifactual "partial images" of the object as if it actually had different locations along the phase encoding direction. Note that it does not matter which direction the object is moving or which gradient is on; if the object moves along the same axis as the gradient (while it is on), then the phase of its MDM vectors will be altered, and its phase encoding coordinates will be changed. Fig. 16.1 illustrates these two types of motion artifact.

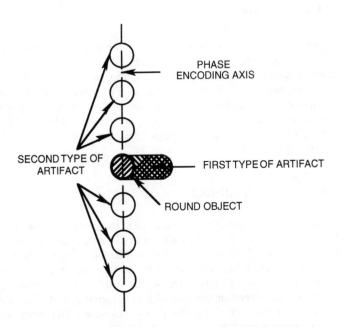

FIG. 16.1- TWO TYPES OF MOTION ARTIFACT
The round object moves to the right creating a blur (first type of artifact); while false images or "ghosts" of the object appear along the phase encoding axis (second type of artifact). Note that the ghosts occur symmetrically on both sides of the horizontal axis.

Periodic Motion

Periodic motion is seen with diaphragmatic movement, pulsating vessels, pulsating CSF, etc. If the motion is periodic, that is, if the object oscillates, then we get what is known as "ghosts", which are multiple false images of the object aligned along the phase encoding direction. Of course, this is an application of the second type of motion artifact described above. It turns out that the spacing between ghosts is directly proportional to the number of signal averages, the TR and the frequency of the periodic motion. Hence, for example, if a given pulse sequence yields a certain distance between ghosts, then doubling either the TR, the number of averages or the frequency of the motion will double the space between the ghosts (fig. 16.2).

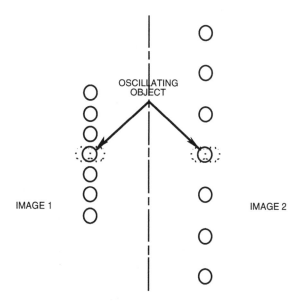

FIG. 16.2- TWO IMAGES SHOWING DIFFERENT "GHOST FREQUENCIES"
In both images, the phase encoding axis is vertical. In image 2, the spacing between the ghosts is twice that of image 1, and either the TR, or the number of signal averages, or the frequency of oscillation of the moving object is double that of image 1.

This concept has immediate practical consequences. For example, when we image the abdomen, the pulsating aorta may produce ghosts of itself in the phase encoding axis, which can mimic high signal intensity lesions in the liver. We may want to alter the TR or number of signal averages in order to place the ghosts in different positions so as not to cause confusion in the diagnostic interpretation.

Flowing Blood

In addition to producing the motion artifacts discussed in the previous section, flowing blood also has a profound effect on the signal intensity of the vessel that is being imaged. The appearance of flowing blood on MR images can be divided into two major categories on the basis of the physical principles: (1) "time-of-flight" phenomena and (2) phase related phenomena. We will consider each of these separately.

Time-of-Flight Phenomena

There are two types of time-of-flight phenomena. One produces vascular images of low signal intensity, and the other produces vascular images of high signal intensity.

Low Signal Type

This is probably the most significant of the phenomena and accounts for the appearance of rapidly moving blood on most MR spin-echo images. Remember that in a spin-echo sequence, there is a 90° RF pulse followed by a series of 180° pulses. Remember also that the tissue affected by these RF pulses is selected by the slice select gradient. Now if blood is rapidly moving within the selected slice, there will be some blood cells traveling so fast that they will exit the slice before they receive both RF pulses. Specifically, if the protons in these moving blood cells receive a 90° pulse, and then exit the region of excitation (selected slice) before receiving the 180° RF pulse in that cycle, they will simply be flipped 90°. Now with the next *slice selection*, they will again be subjected to a 90° RF pulse. (Remember that all this is occurring during one repetition-c.f. fig. 13.2.) But that will result in a total flip of 180°. And we must remember from chapter 3 that if the vectors are in a 180° position, they will not yield a signal (fig. 16.3). Therefore, rapidly moving blood will usually yield a **signal void** (no signal) on standard spin-echo pulse sequences.

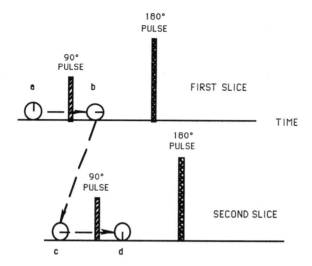

**FIG. 16.3- MDM VECTORS ON A MOVING BLOOD CELL DURING
2 SUCCESSIVE SLICE SELECTIONS**
In position a, the blood cell is in the 1st slice prior to the RF pulse (vector at 12:00). In position b, the blood cell has been subjected to a 90° RF pulse (vector now at 3:00). Then the blood cell exits the first slice before the 180° RF pulse, and enters the region for the 2nd slice (position c- vector still at 3:00). It is then subjected to another 90° pulse as the second slice is excited (position d). This results in a net vector flip of 180° (vector now at 6:00). Now the blood cell vectors have no signal.

High Signal Type

This phenomenon is sometimes called "flow related enhancement" and is seen with vessels that course perpendicular to the plane of the images in a given pulse sequence.

Let us begin by considering a vessel as it penetrates the *first* slice of a multislice spin-echo sequence from outside the imaging volume. In other words, we are considering the case where the blood is flowing in the same direction as the "slice excitation wave" (i.e., the same direction as the slice select *order*). This is called **"cocurrent flow"**. Remember from chapter 5 that if the TR of a pulse sequence is short enough relative to the T1 relaxation times of the tissues, then the pulse sequence will not allow complete vertical recovery of the Mz vector (T1 relaxation) before the next pulse cycle; and if the Mz vertical vector does not return to its original height, then when it is flipped by the next 90° RF pulse, the resultant horizontal Mx vector also will not be as great. Therefore, the resulting signal strength will be less (c.f. fig. 5.2 in chapter 5). This effect is known as "saturation". Of course, in order for this to be the case, the pulse cycle must be applied to the same tissue multiple times. In other words, we must be dealing with **stationary** tissues. A blood cell, however, is not stationary, and when it enters the first slice it has no history of having been flipped. Hence it will possess a maximum Mz vector and therefore yield a maximum Mx vector when it is flipped by the 90° RF pulse. We speak of this situation for the blood cell as being "unsaturated". Therefore, when the blood cell enters the first slice, its unsaturated signal will be relatively stronger than the saturated stationary tissues already in that slice (fig. 16.4).

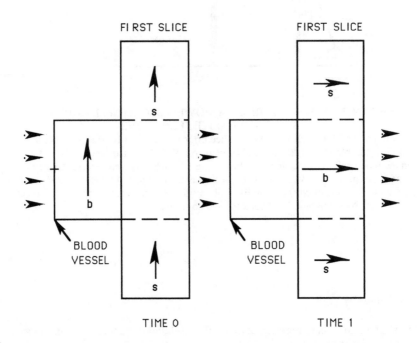

FIG. 16.4- BLOOD VESSEL PENETRATING THE FIRST SLICE

The groups of 4 arrowheads indicate the direction of blood flow (horizontal). "**b**" indicates the blood cell MDM vectors, and "**s**" indicates the stationary tissues' MDM vectors. TIME 0 is in the middle of the pulse sequence, but just before the next 90° RF pulse. At TIME 0, the blood cell has not yet entered the first slice. Note that the Mz vector of the blood cell is greater than that of the stationary tissues, because, unlike the stationary vectors, the blood cell vectors have never been flipped. At TIME 1, the blood cell has entered the slice, and the 90° RF pulse has been applied. Note that the resultant signal is greater for the blood cell than for the stationary tissues, because the blood cell's Mz vector was greater than the stationary tissues' Mz vector prior to the 90° flip.

Now as the blood cell penetrates other slices deeper in the imaging volume, it tends to become saturated. This is because the blood cell will be subjected to additional RF pulses for each excited slice that it enters, and then its Mz will be diminished for exactly the same reasons as described above for the stationary tissues (fig. 16.5). However, the greater the velocity of the blood cell, the more it retains its state of unsaturation as it penetrates the imaging volume, because it tends to out-distance the slice excitation wave which it is "racing".

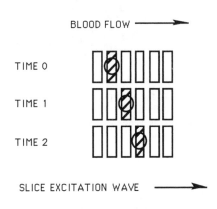

FIG. 16.5- COCURRENT FLOW

Blood flow and slice excitation wave are in the same direction. At each point in time, the blood cell (circle) is in the same slice that is being excited (hatched slice). Hence the cell receives 3 sets of RF pulses, and its MDM vectors tend to become saturated.

So in essence, when blood is flowing cocurrently, its signal will be strongest the closer it is to the first slice and the faster it is flowing. Now let us take this one step further. If laminar flow is present, (cf. p. 135) then the fastest moving blood is found in the center of the vessel. Therefore, the effects of unsaturated blood vs. saturated stationary tissues will be seen to the greatest extent in the center of the vessel. We see that this results in "doughnuts" whose holes are bright signals that decrease in diameter as the blood penetrates into deeper slices (fig. 16.6).

Now if blood is moving opposite to or against the direction of the slice excitation wave (**"countercurrent flow"**), then we tend to see brighter signal intensities at all slice levels than with cocurrent flow. This is partly explained by the following: once the blood cell has passed through an excited slice, it will not encounter another excited slice until the next pulse cycle and therefore, it will experience RF pulses less frequently than in the cocurrent situation. Hence the blood cells in the countercurrent example will be less saturated and will therefore yield a greater signal (fig. 16.7).

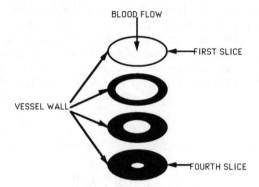

FIG. 16.6- FLOW-RELATED ENHANCEMENT

Blood is flowing perpendicular to the slice plane and is going in the same direction as the slice excitation wave. Note that the largest diameter of increased intensity is in the first slice, and it progressively decreases as deeper slices are imaged.

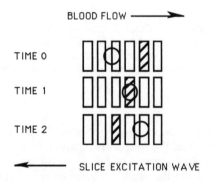

FIG. 16.7- COUNTERCURRENT FLOW

Blood flow and slice excitation wave are in the opposite direction. At TIME 0, the blood cell is entering the 3rd slice from our left, and the 2nd slice from our right is selected (excited). At TIME 1, the blood cell is now in the slice that is selected and experiences an RF pulse. At TIME 2, the blood cell continues traveling to the right, while the slice excitation wave progresses to the left. The two will not encounter each other again at least until the next pulse cycle, and possibly not until the cell is re-circulated (approximately 10-15 sec.). Hence the cell receives fewer RF pulses and would therefore be less saturated than in the cocurrent example.

In the last chapter, we mentioned the fact that flowing blood usually has a high signal intensity on fast scans. We are now able to offer at least a partial explanation of that phenomenon. With fast scans, there is no 180° refocusing pulse, the TE is much shorter, and therefore the blood cell does not get a chance to "escape" to the next slice before its signal is measured. In fact, there is no "next slice" until all the data for the current slice has been obtained. Hence low signal time-of-flight considerations, which usually play an important role in producing a signal void in spin-echo sequences, do not apply to fast scanning. Also, flow-related enhancement (high signal time-of-flight) plays a major role because its effect tends to be seen in the first slice; and with fast scanning, every slice is a first slice (because we do not use a multi-slice technique, as described above). In other words, the blood cell MDM vectors do not get as easily saturated as they do in a spin-echo multi-slice technique. These ideas will be crucial in our discussion of magnetic resonance angiography, in the next chapter.

Phase-Related Phenomena

In chapter 11, we illustrated two sine waves (with the same frequency) out of phase by 60° (fig. 11.2). If those sine waves are out of phase by 180°, and if we add them together, then they completely cancel each other out, and we get no signal (fig. 16.8). Mathematically, these two signals can be represented by $\sin(x)$ and $\sin(x+180°)$. And in fact, by trigonometric identities, $\sin(x+180°) = -\sin(x)$. Therefore, $\sin(x) + \sin(x+180°) = \sin(x) - \sin(x) = 0$, which is equivalent to no signal. This is the process of **dephasing**.

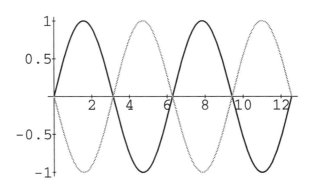

FIG. 16.8- SINE WAVE CANCELLATION
Note that each sine wave is the mirror image of the other reflected across the x axis. If the two curves are added, then the y values for each wave cancel each other out at each point on the x axis, and the result will be no curve at all, i.e., no signal.

However, at the other end of the spectrum, if there is *no* phase shift, then when the two signals are added, the result is a signal whose maximum amplitude is larger than either of the two component signals (and in fact is equal to the sum of the maximum amplitude of each component wave). This is the process of **rephasing.** Hence we have a continuum: as the phase is shifted from 0° to 180°, we gradually achieve more and more dephasing; and as the phase continues from 180° to 360°, we gradually return to a greater degree of rephasing. Fig. 16.9 illustrates the gradual process of dephasing.

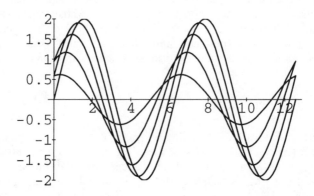

FIG. 16.9- ILLUSTRATION OF GRADUAL DEPHASING
Here are 5 sine curves- all of the same frequency. Each curve represents the sum of 2 sine curves of identical frequency with a phase shift between them. The phase shifts vary in 18° increments from 0° (no phase shift) in the highest amplitude curve to 144° in the lowest amplitude curve. Note the gradual flattening of the curves (decreased signal intensity) as dephasing proceeds on the continuum from 0° to 180°. (At 180°, there is no curve, as we saw above.)

Here is an important corollary:

> If a collection of spins is initially in phase, then **any** change in phase in **any** of the spins will produce a net **decrease** in the total signal.

This is because if they start out in phase, they are already at 0° (or 360°), which is at the maximum end of the continuum, and any change in phase must shift towards the 180° end of the continuum, which is in the dephasing direction as explained above.

Now there are two types of phase-related phenomena: effects related to turbulence and effects related to even and odd echoes in a multiple spin-echo sequence.

Turbulence

When blood flows rapidly through a relatively narrow caliber vessel, it exhibits what is known as "laminar flow". This means that the blood flows in "layers", where the inner-most layer moves at the highest velocity, and the outer-most layer moves at the lowest velocity. Actually, these layers are really *cylinders* of flowing blood within the blood vessel (fig. 16.10).

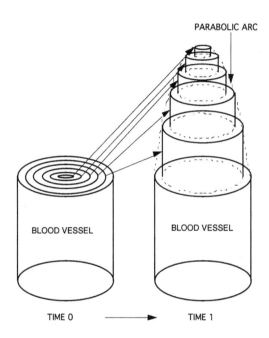

PARABOLIC ARC

BLOOD VESSEL

BLOOD VESSEL

TIME 0 ⟶ TIME 1

FIG. 16.10- LAMINAR FLOW

At time 0, we show a hypothetical static blood vessel prior to laminar flow. At time 1, after a certain period of time, we see that the central-most cylinder of blood has traveled the furthest, and the peripheral-most cylinder has traveled the least. The dashed line that connects the margins of these advancing cylinders of blood is a parabola. For simplicity, we have only illustrated six cylinders. In reality, there would be a large number of extremely thin cylinders.

However, when blood flows slowly through a relatively larger vessel, then laminar flow does not occur, and instead, there is more random motion of the blood cells. This random movement of spinning MDM vectors produces phase shifts among the different moving cells (because they are moving through magnetic gradients), and according to the corollary stated above, this will produce dephasing and a reduction in signal. Therefore, with turbulent flow, we often see a signal void.

Even and Odd Echo Effects

Consider a spin-echo with four echoes whose TE values are 20, 40, 60 and 80 milliseconds. The TE's of 20 mS and 60 mS are the 1st and 3rd echoes respectively, whereas the TE's of 40 mS and 80 mS are the 2nd and 4th echoes respectively. Hence the signals measured at 20 and 60 mS are considered the *odd* echoes, whereas those measured at 40 and 80 mS are considered the *even* echoes. It turns out that with laminar blood flow, there tends to be **de**phasing of the blood cell MDM vectors on the odd echoes and **re**phasing on the even echoes. Hence the vascular structures would appear of low signal intensity on the odd echo images and high signal intensity on the even echo images. We cannot go into the exact cause of this phenomenon, but it has something to do with the fact that there is a parabolic relationship of the blood cell velocity from the center to the periphery of the vessel (fig. 16.10). This imparts a pattern of either diverging or converging phase changes among the different "cylinders" of blood flow. The interaction of this phenomenon with the 180° refocusing pulses that occur for each echo produces the alternating effect of dephasing and rephasing. For a more complete explanation, the reader is referred to Dr. Bradley's article on flow phenomena in the *American Journal of Roentgenology.*[*]

Note that these phenomena occur only when a *symmetrical* multi-echo is employed, i.e., a multi-echo where the time interval is constant between two successive echoes. An example is the situation described above, where the TE values were 20, 40, 60 and 80 mS. Another example would be 30, 60, 90 and 120, or just 40 and 80 for a double echo. (Note that the standard TE 20/80 double echo is *not* an example of a symmetrical multi-echo, because the time interval from 0 to 20 mS is not equal to that between 20 and 80 mS.) We can sort of understand intuitively why this must be the case, for if one echo is associated with dephasing and the next with rephasing, we would expect the time interval to be the same in order to "toggle" back and forth between these two opposing states. It is analogous to our discussion in chapter 6 of how the 180° refocusing pulse works.

Note that although we have considered each flow phenomenon separately, it would be an over-simplification to think that we can always predict the intensity of flowing blood, for we could have more than one of these phenomena applying at the same time. For example, if blood is moving rapidly, then low signal time-of-flight considerations will predominate, and there will be no flow-related enhancement- simply a flow-void (no signal).

---

[*] Bradley WG. Flow phenomena in MR imaging. *AJR* 1988; 150: 983-993.

Summary of Flow Phenomena

Decreased Intravascular Signal Intensity

(1) **Time-of-flight**–seen with rapidly moving blood.
(2) **Odd echo dephasing**–must have symmetric multi-echoes; can be seen in any plane.

Increased Intravascular Signal Intensity

(1) **Even echo rephasing**–must have symmetric multi-echoes; can be seen in any plane.
(2) **Time-of-flight (flow-related enhancement)**–seen with slower flowing blood in the plane perpendicular to the direction of the blood flow.

Methods to Combat Motion Artifacts

In this section, we will discuss four common devices used to reduce the effects of motion artifact.

Pre-saturation

Pre-saturation derives its greatest use in reducing the motion artifact secondary to vascular pulsation. Consider a standard spin-echo sequence. Prior to the application of the usual 90° pulse initiating the spin-echo pulse cycle, an extra 90° pulse is applied to that volume of tissue *not* within the image volume. In other words, for this additional 90° pulse, the frequency components and the slice select gradient are modified in order to select the tissue that is not within the proposed region of imaging. Now, if blood cells from this pre-selected region enter the image volume, their vectors will already have been flipped 90° by this extra RF pulse; and then when the 2nd 90° pulse in the pulse cycle is applied, the blood cell vectors will become flipped a full 180°, and will therefore yield no signal. However, the stationary tissues within the image volume will have been subjected to only one of the 90° pulses, and therefore they will have a signal (fig. 16.11).

By decreasing the signal of moving blood, this method reduces the intensity of the blur and ghost artifacts that may result due to normal blood flow. One may wonder why all this is necessary, since time-of-flight phenomena will automatically produce a flow void. But remember that time-of-flight phenomena apply only to rapidly moving blood, and even in a high flow vessel, there may be components to the flow which do not move so rapidly.

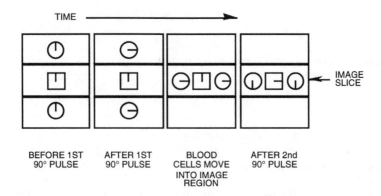

FIG. 16.11- PRE-SATURATION

A stack of 3 slices is shown at each of 4 points in time. The middle slice is the image region. The circles represent blood cells, and the squares are stationary tissues in the image slice. Before the 1st 90° pulse, no vectors are flipped (all vector positions are at 12:00); after the 1st 90° pulse, only the outer slices are selected (vector positions are now at 3:00 in the outer slices but remain at 12:00 in the middle slice); after the 2nd 90° pulse, only the image slice is selected, but the blood cell and stationary tissues' vectors are flipped 90° (vector positions are at 6:00 for the blood cells and 3:00 for the stationary tissues). The blood cell vectors result in a total flip of 180° and therefore have no signal, whereas the stationary tissues result in only a 90° flip and therefore have a signal.

In summary, the pulse cycle for a pre-saturation spin echo is:

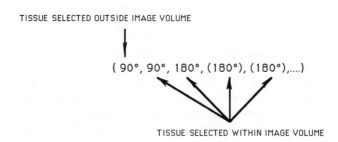

Cardiac Gating

The following discussion applies only to spin-echo pulse sequences. Cardiac gating can be used to control vascular pulsation artifacts and the principle is fairly simple: the TR of the pulse cycle is forced to be equal to the time interval between heart beats. The patient is monitored, and each pulse cycle is triggered by a given event in the cardiac cycle-usually the R wave of the QRS complex of the EKG. This ensures that every time a given slice location is selected, the data will be obtained at the same point in the cardiac cycle, and therefore the position of the contracting walls of the heart will also be the same, and hence the effect of motion will be minimized (fig. 16.12).

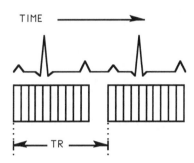

FIG. 16.12- CARDIAC GATING

Two contiguous pulse cycles are shown in a 10 slice acquisition. Each of the 2 sets of rectangles represents the sequential excitation of the 10 slices during the TR for each pulse cycle; and the corresponding EKG events are correlated in time with them. Note how any given slice number lines up with the same point in the EKG in both of the pulse cycles. For example, slice number 4 lines up with the Q wave. (Note also that for the sake of graphic demonstration, we did not use the R wave to trigger the pulse cycle.)

We are not saying that the ventricular walls will be in the same position for all the different slices; in fact, they will be in a different position for each slice number. However, if we choose a slice number, the cardiac position for that slice number will be the same (theoretically) for each successive TR (i.e., for each pulse cycle). In this text, we will not be covering the more complex topic of gating for the purpose of examining the heart in different phases of the cardiac cycle.

Respiratory Ordered Phase Encoding

It may seem to the reader that we ought to be able to do respiratory gating in the same fashion that we discussed for cardiac gating. However, as with cardiac gating, the TR would have to be equal to the time interval between respirations. Since most people breathe approximately 12 times per minute, this would require a TR of 5 seconds or 5000 mS, which would yield an examination time that is unacceptable. However, there exists a neat device known as "respiratory ordered phase encoding" ("ROPE"). Once again, remember that in a standard 2DFT pulse sequence, the phase encoding steps are applied from -180° to +180° in increments which depend on the matrix size. What ROPE does is to *rearrange* the order of the phase encoding steps so that they correlate with respiratory motion in a manner more suited to reducing the motion artifact due to breathing. In other words, ROPE is simply a permutation of the usual phase encoding steps- the same steps are obtained, but simply in a different order; and hence the time of the examination is not appreciably altered.

It turns out that those phase encoding "rows" nearest the edges of the matrix (i.e., those closest to -180° and +180°) are the most sensitive in determining spatial resolution. This is a direct corollary of the attributes of k-space (p. 92). Out of this emerges a ROPE strategy: apply those important "edge of the matrix" phase encoding steps to that portion of the respiratory cycle where the diaphragms move the least; and likewise, apply the more central phase encoding steps (those around 0° phase encoding) to the region of the respiratory cycle where the diaphragms move the most. Fig. 16.13 illustrates this process for a simple matrix.

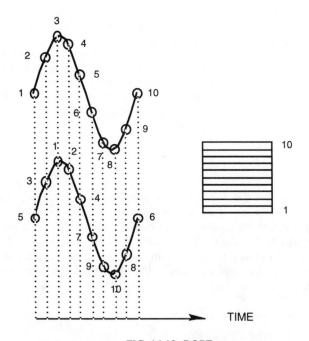

FIG. 16.13- ROPE
The top curve represents 1 respiratory cycle with normal sequential phase encoding, and the bottom represents 1 respiratory cycle with ROPE. The square on the right shows 10 horizontal phase encoding steps in a slice matrix. The numbers on the curves correspond to the 10 rows of the matrix. In the non-ROPE curve, phase encoding proceeds sequentially from the bottom to the top rows of the matrix. But in the ROPE sequence, a different permutation is used such that the edges of the matrix are encoded at the highest and lowest points of diaphragmatic excursion, i.e., where the diaphragms move the least.

For a normal 2DFT acquisition with 10 phase steps, the phase encoding sequence would be:

$$\{-180°, -144°, -108°, -72°, -36°, 0°, +36°, +72°, +108°, +144°\}.$$

For the ROPE example in fig. 16.13, the sequence is:

$$\{-36°, -108°, -180°, -144°, -72°, +36°, +108°, +144°, +72°, 0°\}.$$

These two permutations of phase encoding steps correspond respectively to the two sequences of row numbers of the matrix shown in fig. 16.13:

$$\{1,2,3,4,5,6,7,8,9,10\} \text{ and } \{5,3,1,2,4,7,9,10,8,6\}.$$

In practical usage, a transducer is applied to the patient to measure abdominal excursion during respiration, and then the ordering of the phase encoding steps is determined on that basis. Of course, ROPE is not perfect, since the effects of motion are modified–not eliminated. In actual practice, some ROPE sequences work beautifully, whereas others yield images that appear to have as much motion artifact as if ROPE were never used. Incidentally, one of the major vendors, GE Medical (Milwaukee), calls their version of ROPE "the Exorcist"™, because it eliminates ghosts, of course.

Gradient Moment Nulling

Gradient moment nulling (GMN) attempts to reduce motion artifacts with the use of gradients only. Remember that one of the main components of motion artifact is due to the phase changes that result from an object moving in the direction of a gradient. What gradient moment nulling does is to modify the frequency and slice select gradients when they are applied so that the effects of phase shift due to motion become nullified. Technically, this is accomplished by first applying the gradient as it would normally be applied, then applying a negative gradient of twice the strength, and finally re-applying the original positive gradient (fig. 16.14).

GRADIENT AMPLITUDE

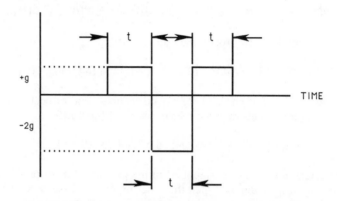

FIG. 16.14- GRADIENT CONFIGURATION FOR GMN
There are 3 "lobes" to this gradient. Each is applied for a time t. The first and third are positive, and the middle is negative and double the amplitude (slope) of the first and third.

In previous discussions, we have considered the gradient as a sloped line whose x axis is distance and whose y axis is magnetic field strength. Let us now consider just one spinning MDM vector moving at a constant velocity along the direction of an increasing gradient. According to the Larmor equation, the frequency of this spinning vector will increase as it travels along the line of the gradient. Now because the strength of the magnetic field increases linearly, so will the frequency of the MDM vector. And since it is traveling at a constant velocity, its frequency will also increase linearly with time. Fig. 16.15 below shows a graph of the frequency of the MDM vector spin vs. time as it experiences the three components of the GMN gradient.

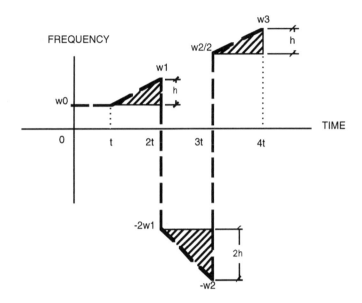

FIG. 16.15 GRAPH OF MDM FREQUENCY vs. TIME DURING GMN
We consider an MDM with an initial frequency of w0 in a clockwise direction. The heavy dashed line represents the graph of its frequency vs. time while it moves at constant velocity during the 3 lobes of the GMN gradient. (Note that the relative value of each frequency is its distance from the TIME axis.) At time t, the 1st positive lobe is applied. At time 2t, the frequency has increased to w1. Then the negative lobe is applied at double the strength. This makes it spin twice as fast *counter*-clockwise; so now the frequency is immediately changed to -2w1. At time 3t, its counter-clockwise frequency has increased to -w2. Now the 3rd lobe is applied exactly like the 1st. This immediately reverses the direction of the spin back to clockwise and cuts the frequency in half, so that it is now w2/2. Note that the vertical leg of the triangle beneath the TIME axis is twice that of each of the 2 triangles above the axis (because the lobe between t and 2t, and the lobe between 3t and 4t, is half the strength as the lobe between 2t and 3t); and the horizontal legs of all the triangles are equal (because the duration of time is the same for each lobe of the gradient). Therefore the combined area of the 2 triangles above the TIME axis equals the area of the triangle below it, and hence their total sum is 0. Hence the net angular displacement, or *phase shift* is also 0 (th + th - t2h = th + th - 2th = 0).

Now as we have said before, phase shift is frequency times time. However, since the MDM vector is moving, we cannot simply multiply frequency times time to determine its resultant phase shift. This is because its frequency is constantly changing. On the other hand, calculus teaches us that we can calculate the phase shift simply by taking the area under the frequency-time curves in fig. 16.15. Considering the area beneath the x axis to be negative, we see that the triangular areas all add up to 0, which of course means that there is no resultant phase shift. Hence, anytime we wish to apply a gradient where there are moving spins, we can use the GMN technique (theoretically) to ensure that there are no resultant phase shifts due to motion through that gradient.

The reader may be more familiar with GMN under other names: MAST™(Motion Artifact Suppression Technique–Picker Intl., Cleveland) and "flow compensation"™ (GE Medical, Milwaukee).

Note that when GMN is used, there is very little of the usual flow void even in rapidly moving blood.

The reader should beware that as with the other techniques that we discussed, GMN is not perfect. For example, if the motion is not linear, then the gradient configuration described above will not apply. However, the reader should also note that some applications of GMN, such as MAST, are designed to accommodate higher orders of motion, such as acceleration.

17
Magnetic Resonance Angiography (MRA)

There are two major approaches to producing an MRA image: (1) utilizing the principle of time-of-flight; and (2) utilizing phase contrast techniques.

Time-of-Flight (TOF)

With this technique, the blood vessels are visualized using a standard fast scan or gradient echo sequence. This yields a bright signal for moving blood because of saturation phenomena, as we discussed on p. 128, an example of flow related enhancement. However, there are many other tissues that also appear as relatively high signal intensities on fast scan images. Therefore, the goal is to *selectively* image the vascular structures. This is accomplished using the "maximum intensity projection" (MIP) algorithm. Here is the way it works. Once the image volume[*] is obtained, the computer scans the data by examining the signal intensity in each slice corresponding to the coordinates of each pixel in the plane in which the projection is being obtained. In other words, it is as if the computer "peers" through a channel of data for each pixel in the projection axis. It then records in that coordinate location the brightest intensity encountered within that channel of data (fig. 17.1).

The computer does this for pixel position (1,1), (1,2), etc., until it finishes up with position (256,256). In this fashion, we wind up with a coronal image representing a **projection** of the image data in all the slices. Because the vascular structures tend to be the brightest tissues on a fast scan image, they will be favored on the final projection, i.e., if there are other less bright tissues along the same line of projection as a vessel, they will not be recorded, and the vessel will therefore not be obscured.

---

[*] Remember that the term "image volume" simply refers to the MR slices all stacked one on top of the other to obtain a rectangular solid.

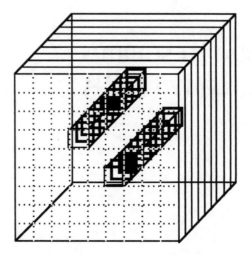

FIG. 17.1- MIP ALGORITHM FOR 2 PIXELS IN THE CORONAL PLANE
The large block represents an image volume with a fictitious 9 x 9 matrix with 10 thin but gapped coronal slices. The computer is considering the 2 channels of data at the pixel positions (4,4) and (6,6). The stacks of small thick-lined squares represent the pixels at these two positions for each of the ten slices. Note that in the channel for position (4,4), the pixel in slice number 6 from the front is darkened to show that it has the highest signal intensity of the pixels in the channel; whereas in the (6,6) channel it is the pixel in slice number 3 that has the highest signal intensity. Each of these signal intensities is then recorded at pixel locations (4,4) and (6,6) respectively in the final image.

It is interesting that the MIP algorithm sort of reverses the effects of cross-sectional imaging. It projects into one plane the information that is present on multiple planes. In other words, it is as if we were constructing a contact radiograph from tomographic slices. But this is exactly what we want, for it is difficult to image a meandering vessel in a single plane.

3DFT vs. 2DFT Techniques

The MIP algorithm can be used for either a 2DFT or a 3DFT MRA sequence exactly as described in chapter 14. There are pros and cons for the use of each technique. For example, the 3DFT technique may be less suitable than the 2DFT technique for imaging slowly flowing blood. This is because the thick slab of the 3DFT technique will allow slowly moving blood to be exposed to more RF pulses and become relatively more saturated, and hence, more difficult to distinguish from the stationary tissues. However, since a 2DFT sequence employs multiple thin slices, there is less time for the blood to become saturated before exiting and flowing into the next slice. So blood would have a higher signal intensity relative to stationary tissues with the 2DFT sequence.

Also, if all other things are equal, the 3DFT technique is better for imaging tortuous vessels. Once blood has penetrated a thick slab in a 3DFT sequence, its saturation characteristics are not affected by the direction in which it moves, since the RF pulses affect the entire slab On the other hand, effective visualization of blood flow with the 2DFT technique depends on movement of the blood in a direction perpendicular to the plane of the slices. It is as if the thick slab in the 3DFT technique gives the blood more room to move around in comparison to the multiple thin slices of a 2DFT acquisition.

Strategy for Slow Flow with the 3DFT Technique

As described above, blood flowing slowly through a 3DFT slab will have diminished signal intensity because of increasing saturation. Therefore, to optimize the images in this situation, we should use parameters that reduce saturation as much as possible. The factors we can readily alter that affect saturation are TR and flip angle. As we increase the TR, we allow more time for recovery of the longitudinal Mz vector, and hence increase the signal obtained on subsequent flips; hence we reduce saturation of the blood. Also, if we decrease the flip angle, there is less distance for the Mz vector to travel to completely recover; so this also reduces blood saturation. Therefore, to optimize vascular visualization on a 3DFT sequence when there is slow flow, we should increase the TR and/or decrease the flip angle.

Magnetic Transfer Contrast (MTC)

"Magnetic transfer contrast" is a term used to describe the phenomenon whereby magnetization of hydrogen MDM vectors in bound water molecules transfer their magnetization to the hydrogen vectors of nearby *unbound* water molecules. By "bound" water molecules, we mean water molecules chemically bound to macromolecular substances, such as the brain. Since magnetization is transferred, the relaxation properties of the recipient MDM vectors become changed. Hence MTC can be thought of as a process complicating T1 and T2 relaxation by altering the relaxation characteristics of free water molecules adjacent to bound water molecules. More specifically, as a result of MTC, the MDM vectors receiving the transferred magnetization acquire greater saturation than those vectors not partaking in the MTC process.

Let us see how this process can be applied to intracranial MRA to improve contrast between flowing blood and background tissues. In this situation, extravascular water bears a close proximity to the bound water of brain tissue. Hence, it will suffer the effects of MTC and become relatively saturated. However, intravascular flowing blood consists almost exclusively of unbound water with no nearby bound water to provide MTC. Hence, intravascular blood will be relatively less saturated and therefore will have a greater signal intensity than the extravascular unbound water of the background tissues. More simply, if tissue A is subjected to the MTC phenomenon, and tissue B is not, then tissue A will become more saturated than B hence increasing the contrast of B relative to A.

Because of the neighboring macromolecular substances, bound water will have a different precession frequency from unbound water. In actual practice, therefore, the bound water molecules are selectively pulsed when MTC is invoked in an MRA sequence.

Phase Contrast MRA

This method is more complex than time-of-flight. With time-of-flight MRA, we visualized the vascular structures by using a fast scan (gradient echo scan) to make them bright, and then we used MIP to distinguish them from other bright objects. Phase contrast MRA makes use of a different principle to "label" the blood vessels: phase. In order to avoid confusion, for what follows, we will distinguish *axis* from *direction* in accordance with our definitions in the section on vectors: we will use "axis" to refer to the orthogonality of the flow (i.e., whether it is along the x, y or z axis); and we will use "direction" to refer to which way it is flowing along a particular axis.

Remember from p. 125 that whenever anything moves along the axis of an applied gradient, the phase of the spinning vectors in that object become altered relative to stationary objects. Hence we have a method for selectively labeling blood vessels.

In order to make this work, a bipolar gradient is used. Bipolar gradients are gradients which are positive in one direction for a period of time, and then negative in the opposite direction for the same period of time and amplitude fig. 17.2 (or negative first and then positive).

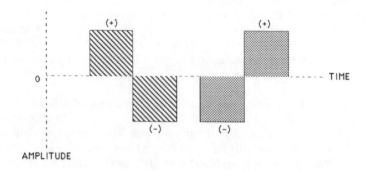

FIG. 17.2- BIPOLAR GRADIENTS

They have the effect of changing the phase only on moving objects. This is because the positive and negative lobes of the gradient cancel each other's phase changes out for stationary objects; but since the moving object acquires its own phase change, it will be left with a residual phase alteration relative to stationary objects. This phase alteration (ϕ) is a function of the gyro magnetic ratio (γ), the velocity of the moving blood particles (V), the time interval between the lobes of the bipolar gradient (T) and the area of each gradient lobe (A): $\phi = \gamma VTA^{*}$.

In practice, we first choose the axis along which we wish to apply the label. Then we obtain two sequences with a bipolar gradient applied along this axis. In one sequence, the gradient goes from positive to negative, and in the other, it goes from negative to positive. This yields zero phase change for the stationary objects in both sequences, a positive phase change for the moving blood in one sequence, and an equal but opposite negative phase change for moving blood in the other sequence. We then subtract one of these sequences from the other, pixel by pixel. This has the effect of canceling any acquired background phase changes (of stationary objects) as well as heightening the phase shift of the moving blood (because a positive minus a negative gives *two* positives).

The MR scanner determines the phase change for each pixel, and of course those pixels corresponding to the location of moving blood will have greater phase shifts than the stationary tissues. That is how the blood vessels become labeled. Next we need a mapping device to translate the moving blood into relative densities. This is done basically by one of two methods, known as "phase difference" and "complex difference" processing

Phase Difference

The phase difference method linearly maps the phase shift angle into a signal intensity, and hence density, so that 0° phase shift (stationary tissues) is medium gray, objects moving in one direction along the axis of the bipolar gradient are bright, and objects moving in the opposite direction along the axis of the bipolar gradient are dark. For example, a shift of +30° (+p/6) would be brighter than a shift of +15° (+p/12); and a shift of -30° (-p/6) would be darker than a shift of -15° (-p/12). This method therefore has the advantage of indicating the direction of blood flow in a vessel.

Complex Difference

The complex difference method maps the pixel density according to the following function: signal intensity = 2M|sin(f)|, where M is the magnetization in the transverse plane, and f is the angular amount of the phase shift. In this case, since the brightness of the signal depends on a sine function, the map is no longer linear. Also, even though the sine function changes sign, the formula

---

* Note that A = the gradient height times its width, which is actually the amplitude of the gradient times the length of time that it is on.

considers only its absolute value, which nullifies the effect of negative values. Hence, for example, although sin(+30°) = +.5 and sin(-30°) = -.5, |sin(+30°)| = |sin(-30°)| = .5. And since differences in the direction of blood flow are measured in terms of the sign of the phase shift angle, we can see that this method will not indicate blood flow direction.

V_{enc}

One aspect of phase contrast MRA is that the examination is tailored for either rapid or slow flowing blood. Referring to the above formula for phase shift, we see that if V is small (slow moving blood), we can adjust the strength of the gradient (A) to compensate for V and hence maintain a sufficiently large phase change (ϕ) in order to adequately visualize these vessels. This is done by specifying a maximum velocity such that all blood moving at this velocity will map to the brightest density on the final image. This velocity is termed "V_{enc}" because it determines the amplitude of the encoding bipolar gradient. Hence it is the *encoding* velocity. All velocities less than the specified V_{enc} will have their density representations scaled in accordance with that V_{enc}.

Let us now look at the graph of signal intensity vs. velocity for the phase difference method with a given V_{enc} (fig. 17.3).

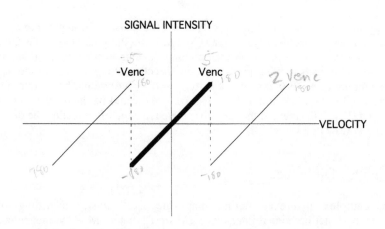

FIG. 17.3 GRAPH OF PHASE DIFFERENCE MAPPING

Remember that with phase difference, signal intensity is a linear function of the phase angle. Also, from the above formula, the phase angle is a linear function of velocity. Therefore, signal intensity is a linear function of velocity. Each diagonal line represents the signal intensities for velocities corresponding to phase shifts from -180° to +180°. Also, the velocities at +180° (or -180°) are multiples of $+V_{enc}$ or $-V_{enc}$ depending on whether we are looking to the right or the left of the y axis. If a phase shift is greater than +180°, for example +180° + 10° (190°), it will be the same as a -180° + 10° and will therefore be mapped as a -170° shift[*]. This explains the cyclical (or periodic) appearance of the graph despite continuously increasing velocities. Also, since positive phase shifts yield bright densities, and negative shifts yield low densities, a velocity slightly greater than V_{enc} (such as the one corresponding to +190°) will be mapped as a low density (a -170° shift). This phenomenon- of blood appearing dark even though its velocity is in a positive direction- represents a form of aliasing, which will occur if the V_{enc} is chosen to be too small.

The graph of signal intensity vs. velocity for complex difference processing is shown in fig. 17.4.

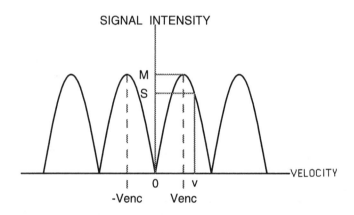

FIG. 17.4- GRAPH OF COMPLEX DIFFERENCE MAPPING
M is the maximum amplitude of the curve, which occurs when the sine function is maximal: at 90°. The corresponding velocity for this 90° phase shift is the Venc. The velocity v is slightly greater than Venc and is mapped at S, a slightly lower amplitude. Hence v is aliased as a decreased density. Note that here, aliasing occurs at 90° shifts, as opposed to 180° shifts for the phase difference method.

---

[*] This is similar to our discussion of aliasing on p. 155.

It is also a cyclic graph, for the same reasons as discussed above. However, since this is an absolute value function, the graph never dips below the x axis, and hence the signal intensity is never negative (i.e., moving blood will always be bright regardless of its direction). Also, multiples of the V_{enc} here are determined by the various peaks of the graph. In this case, if a velocity has a phase shift greater than 90°, it will map to a lower signal intensity than that of the V_{enc}; although it will never map to a negative signal intensity. Hence aliasing for the complex difference method will yield a relatively bright or high density (although less than the maximum) as opposed to aliasing for the phase difference method, which yields a relatively dark or low density, as explained above. Note that with the complex difference method, aliasing occurs with a phase shift greater than 90°, as opposed to 180° for the phase difference method.

Note that regardless of which of the two image processing methods are used, it requires 2 sequences to visualize blood flow along any one axis; and we *only* see blood flow along a single given axis. Therefore, to evaluate flow in all three orthogonal axes, 6 sequences would be necessary. Now there is a neat trick whereby the number of sequences can be cut down to 4, but we will not describe it here.[*]

Speed Image

Finally, we can produce phase contrast studies that portray flow in all 3 axes on the same image with the use of a so called "speed" image. In a speed image, the signal intensity for a given pixel is calculated from the value of the velocity at that pixel location in each of the three axes from the following formula:

$$S = \sqrt{V_x^2 + V_y^2 + V_z^2},$$

where s is the signal intensity for a given pixel location, and v_x, v_y, and v_z represent the velocities in the x, y and z directions at that pixel location. These velocities are obtained from either the phase difference or complex difference processing methods as applied to the pairs of sequences in each of the three axes. Note that the term s is simply a value, which does not preserve any directional information that was present in the velocity vector values; hence s is a scalar (just as "speed" is a scalar term).

---

[*] Those interested in this method can find it in *Clinical Magnetic Resonance Angiography,* by Anderson, et. al. The text refers to the method as "Hadamard multiplexed flow encoding".

Summary

Time-of-flight MRA relies on saturation differences, which in turn is a function of T1 or longitudinal relaxation; whereas phase contrast MRA relies on phase differences of horizontally spinning MDM vectors, in which T2 relaxation is more relevant. Hence we can think of time-of-flight MRA as a T1 or longitudinal process, and phase contrast MRA as a T2 or horizontal process. The following table summarizes some of the differences between the various time-of-flight (TOF) and phase contrast (PC) approaches:

	USES SATURATION	USES PHASE	USES MIP	AXIS SPECIFIC	DIRECTION SPECIFIC	ALL AXES
2D TOF	+	–	+	–	–	+
3D TOF	+	–	+	–	–	+
PC - PD	–	+	–	+	+	–
PC - CD	–	+	–	+	–	–
PC - SPEED	–	+	–	–	–	+

Fig. (17.5) below summarizes the theoretical appearance of blood flowing through a T shaped vessel for the various methods:

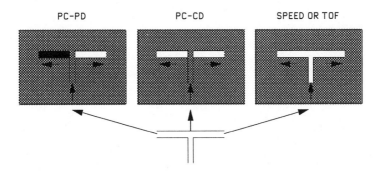

FIG. 17.5- APPEARANCE OF BLOOD IN DIFFERENT MRA TECHNIQUES
"PC" = phase contrast; "PD" = phase difference; "CD" = complex difference. In this case, velocity encoding is along the horizontal axis for both the phase difference and complex difference methods.

18
Aliasing

The author has chosen to create a separate chapter for this topic simply because there is no other chapter that it appropriately fits into. Aliasing (or "wrap-around") is an important artifact that is relatively easy to understand. It is the phenomenon whereby an object that is outside the field of view becomes superimposed over the image, on the side opposite to where it is found. It usually occurs in the phase encoding axis, but can also occur in the frequency axis as well.

Aliasing in the Phase Encoding Axis

If the field of view along the phase encoding axis is smaller than the range of the receiving coil, then aliasing in this axis will occur. Here is what happens. Consider a matrix with 10 phase encoding steps, as we did when we discussed ROPE. Remember that in order to span 360°, the 10 steps had to be separated by a 36 degree interval, ranging from -144° through 0 to +180°. This angular range is illustrated in fig. 18.1.

Fig. 18.2 shows a letter "Y" which is slightly too large for the field of view in the phase encoding direction. Consider the upper "arms" of the "Y". Because of the gradient (which does not stop at the edge of the selected field of view) the parts that project over the top edge of the matrix will be phase shifted an extra 36° beyond 180°.

We can see from fig. 18.1 that this angle of 216° is the same as -144°. Therefore the scanner places that imaging information in the -144° row. That is why the top portions of the arms of the "Y" are "aliased" or "wrapped around" to the bottom row. In other words, the problem is that we have 11 rows to image, but only 10 *different* labels; so therefore 2 rows must have the same label. By the same method of thinking, the stem of the "Y" projects 36° beyond the -144° row, and would hence be phase shifted -180°, which is the same as +180°, and is therefore aliased to the top row.

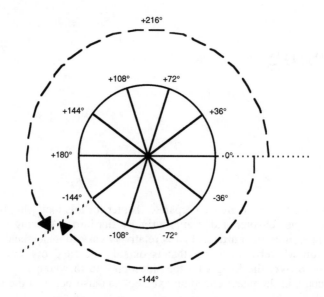

FIG. 18.1- PHASE ENCODING STEPS AS CIRCULAR ANGLES
Note that -144° is a clockwise rotation from 0°; and +216° is a counter-clockwise rotation from 0°. But they are the same angle.

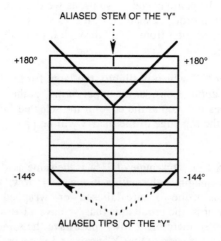

FIG. 18.2- ALIASING
The field of view in the phase encoding direction (vertical) is smaller than the "Y", which is to be imaged.

To combat this artifact, scanners make use of an "anti-aliasing" procedure, which works as follows. The matrix size and the field of view are doubled along the phase encoding axis (fig. 18.3).

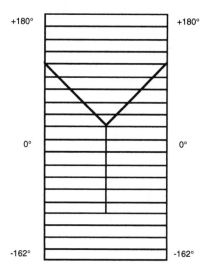

FIG. 18.3- ANTI-ALIASING
The matrix size is doubled from 10 to 20 rows in the phase encoding direction. But the field of view is also doubled in that axis so that the widths of the rows remain the same (pixel size is unchanged). Note that the phase encoding steps are separated by increments of 18° from -162° to +180°.

Now the "Y" fits quite comfortably within the new matrix, and hence each portion of the "Y" is uniquely phase encoded, and therefore no aliasing occurs. In other words, we now have enough different labels for all of the rows in the image. Note that the final image is reconstructed at half the size of the new field of view so that the original field of view is preserved. Note also that the pixel size in the phase encoding direction (width of the rows) is not altered during anti-aliasing, and therefore the resolution of the final image is not disturbed. However, as described so far, the anti-aliasing procedure would take twice as long. Therefore, when anti-aliasing is used, the number of signal averages must be cut in half in order to preserve imaging time. This does not decrease the signal to noise ratio, because the doubled number of rows of data employed in the anti-aliasing procedure exactly compensates for halving the number of signal averages.

Note that some commercial scanners allow the matrix size to vary directly with the field of view in the phase encoding direction, thereby preserving the pixel size in that axis. This can allow anti-aliasing without necessarily doubling the matrix size (and number of repetitions).

Aliasing in the Frequency Encoding Axis

Unlike aliasing in the phase encoding direction, frequency aliasing has nothing to do with the relationship of the field of view to the receiving coil. Remember that the scanner receives the signal by measuring its amplitude for a given instant at fixed intervals in time ("sampling"). Fig. 18.4 below shows a simple sine wave representing an MR signal.

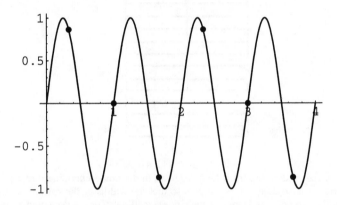

FIG. 18.4- SIMPLE MR SINE WAVE SIGNAL

The tiny circles represent points on the sine wave where low rate sampling has taken place. Except for the first point, the points are all .66 units apart on the time axis. In other words the y coordinate of each point is the amplitude of the signal recorded at equal intervals in time starting at .33 on the time axis.

If we obtain many samples, then the time interval between samples will be short enough to delineate all the peaks and valleys of this curve, and hence we will have an accurate "picture" of it. But suppose that our sampling rate were so low (fig. 18.4) that the time interval between samples was .66 seconds, with the 1st point at .33 seconds (i.e.: at points in time equal to .33, 1, 1.66, 2.33, 3, etc.). Fig. 18.5 below shows the same sine wave superimposed on another sine wave one-half its frequency.

Note that the sampled points on our true signal also fall on the half frequency curve. Since our scanner knows only what it samples, it falsely "assumes" that the signal we are measuring is the one with the lower frequency. Now if the scanner makes this error, then the signal that is recorded will contain lower frequencies than the true signal. Since the edge of our image at the high end of the frequency gradient is encoded with high frequency components, these will be translated into lower frequencies by the sampling error described above. This will effectively take image data from the high frequency part of the frequency axis and map it onto the opposite side, where the low frequency part of the image is found; and hence we get aliasing. In other words: aliasing in the frequency encoding axis occurs when the sampling rate is too low (or too infrequent). This brings us to a technical definition:

The "**Nyquist**" frequency is the frequency beyond which aliasing will occur for a given number of samples. It is equal to one-half of the number of samples.

For example, if there are 512 samples (measurements) in a frequency gradient read-out, then the Nyquist frequency is 256. Or stated another way, if we are to have 256 pixels in the frequency axis, we will need 512 samples during the read (frequency) gradient.

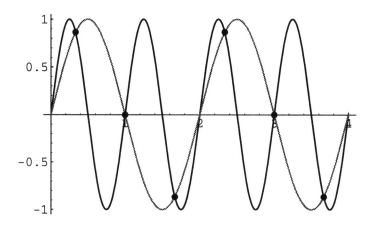

FIG. 18.5- SAMPLING ERROR
The darker curve is the MR signal with its sampling points from fig. 18.4. The sampling points also fall on the gray sine curve, which is half the frequency of the MR signal. The scanner mistakenly thinks that the points belong to the half frequency gray curve.

Incidentally, note an interesting similarity between phase encoding aliasing and frequency encoding aliasing: both involve an ambiguity. With phase encoding, there is more than one row of data assigned to a given phase angle; and with frequency encoding, the sample points belong to two different sine waves.

19
Fat and Water

In this chapter, we will consider some of the important ways that fat and water interact in the MR image. Specifically, we will discuss chemical shift artifacts as well as methods to suppress water and fat. We will find that all but one of the phenomena to be covered are based on one fundamental notion: because of the molecular differences between fat and water, the hydrogen MDM vectors in fat precess 220 cycles per second faster than the hydrogen MDM vectors in water. Hence for a 1.5T magnet, the water MDM's precess at 64,000,000 Hz[*], and the fat MDM's precess at 64,000,**220** Hz. We will see that this simple difference in precession frequency lies at the root of much of what follows in this chapter.

Chemical Shift Artifact

Chemical shift artifacts in MR imaging occur in relation to the **frequency** axis. The common form of chemical shift artifact in spin-echo MR imaging is seen when there is an interface between fat and water (fig. 19.1).

What we see is a light or a dark band at the junction between the fat and the water tissues. Whether the band is light or dark depends on whether the gradient is increasing or decreasing as we move from the fat to the water tissue. In fig. 19.1, we have water on all sides of the fat. A dark band is seen at the left interface, and a bright band is seen at the right; but no band is seen on the top or bottom. The bands are perpendicular to the frequency axis. Here is why we see this phenomenon.

---

[*] Actually, it is not *exactly* 64 million, but we over-simplfy in the interests of demonstration.

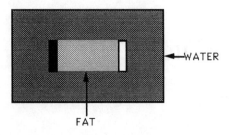

FIG. 19.1- CHEMICAL SHIFT ARTIFACT

In this case, the bright band is on our right, and the dark band is on our left. This tells us (1) that the frequency gradient is horizontal (perpendicular to the bands); and (2) that the frequency gradient increases from left to right.

Fig. 19.2a shows a water-fat-water set of interfaces. The dotted vertical lines show columns of precessing vectors with each column perpendicular to the frequency axis.

Note that even before a gradient is applied, the frequency of the vectors in the fat columns are all precessing 220 Hz faster than the vectors in the water columns. Now, when the frequency (or "read-out") gradient is applied, there will be a gradual increase in the frequency of each column as we move to the right in the increasing direction of the gradient. However, when we reach the region of fat, each column of vectors will jump 220 Hz more than the increased frequency due to the gradient (fig. 19.2b).

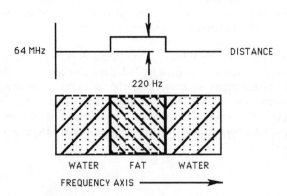

FIG. 19.2a- WATER-FAT-WATER INTERFACE PRIOR TO GRADIENT

Above the blocks of tissues is a graph of frequencies of the columns of MDM vectors vs. distance. Note the 220 Hz jump over the fat tissue. Note also that the graph is horizontal: no frequency gradient has been applied.

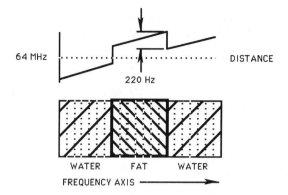

FIG. 19.2b- WATER-FAT-WATER INTERFACE AFTER GRADIENT
The graph of frequency vs. distance is now sloped to reflect the frequency gradient
application, which causes a frequency increase as we move from left to right. However,
there is a discontinuity (jump) in the frequencies at the fat segment.

Later when the image is constructed, this extra 220 Hz for each fat column will
cause the computer to map each of these columns slightly further to the right
relative to water than it would have if these were water columns and not fat.[*]
In other words, the fat region will be shifted to the right relative to the two water
regions (fig. 19.2c).

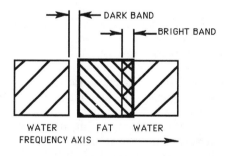

FIG. 19.2c- CHEMICAL SHIFT ARTIFACT
The fat tissue image is shifted slightly to the right, overlapping the water tissue and hence
producing a bright band at the right interface, and a signal void at the left interface.

---

[*] Remember that we use the frequency gradient to mark the location of objects along the
frequency axis, and in fig. 19.2b, the greater the frequency, the more the column will be
mapped to the right.

This will cause a slight overlap of the right margin of the fat tissue with the water tissue just to its right; and hence there will be an **increased** signal (water + fat) in the region of the overlap. And likewise, there will be a region of *no signal* at the left interface of the fat and water- the void resulting from having shifted the fat to the right (fig. 19.2c).

Note that we can establish a rule for relating the direction of the gradient slope to which side of the fat-water interface has which band:

> If we go from water to fat in the same direction that the gradient is increasing, we get a *dark* band; and if we go from fat to water in the same direction that the gradient is increasing, we get a bright band; and vice-versa when the gradient is decreasing.

By looking at our images, we can use this rule to determine which way the gradient slopes (if we want to).

It is also important to realize that the 220 Hz difference between fat and water is subject to the law of the Larmor equation, which means that this frequency difference will be greater on high field strength magnets than on low ones. For example, if 220 Hz is the difference for 1.5T, than on a .75T machine, the frequency difference would be 110 Hz; and therefore the shift would be smaller. Hence chemical shift artifact is more readily seen on high field strength machines.

Method of Dixon

Sometimes the tissue we are imaging contains both fat and water, and we may wish to suppress fat relative to water or vice-versa. The method of Dixon allows us to do this with spin-echo pulse sequences.

First, we must obtain a modified spin-echo pulse sequence. Remember that in a standard spin-echo pulse sequence, the time interval from the 90° RF pulse to the 180° RF pulse is equal to the time interval from the 180° pulse to the measurement of the signal (i.e., the center of the frequency gradient). This is so that the maximum intensity of the rephasing vectors is read at the center of the frequency gradient. But in the Dixon method, the frequency gradient is applied later or slightly earlier than this "optimal" time (fig. 19.3).

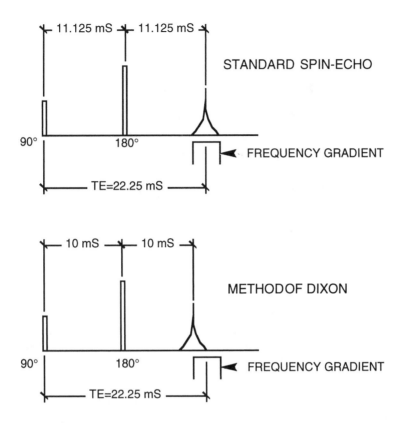

FIG. 19.3- STANDARD SPIN-ECHO CYCLE vs. DIXON METHOD
Note that the standard spin-echo and the Dixon method have the same TE = 22.25 mS. But in the method of Dixon, the peak signal occurs earlier than the signal measurement (frequency gradient) by 2.25 mS; whereas in the standard spin-echo the signal measurement and the peak signal are concurrent. However, note that in **both** cases, the 180° pulse bisects the time between the 90° pulse and the *occurrence* of the signal (not the *measurement* of the signal).

Now remember that water and fat MDM vectors differ in their frequencies by 220 Hz. Consider two one-handed clocks: one is spinning at 64MHz, and the other is spinning at 64MHz + 220 Hz. Imagine that you are traveling around the faces of these clocks at 64MHz. The hand of the "water" clock will appear to you to be stationary (because you are moving around the clock the same speed that it is); but the hand of the "fat" clock is spinning 220 Hz faster than you and will therefore appear to be spinning simply at 220 Hz. This means that its hand will correspond with your position every time it makes a revolution. Now the time it takes for it to make a revolution is the reciprocal of 220 Hz or 1/220, which equals approximately 4.5 mS. Hence you (and the "water" clock) are in phase with the "fat" clock every 4.5 mS. Therefore, if fat and water MDM's start out in phase at time 0, they will again be in phase at approximately every 4.5 mS. This means that they will be 180° apart, or *out of phase* at *half* that time, or approximately every 4.5 mS, *starting* at 2.25 mS (fig. 19.4).

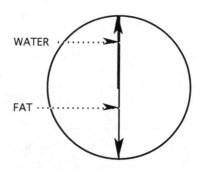

FIG. 19.4- DEPHASING OF WATER AND FAT

If the water and fat vectors were in phase at time 0, then at 2.25 mS, there will be a 180° difference between the water and fat vectors, and there will be dephasing (refer to fig. 16.8 showing sine wave cancellation).

In a standard spin-echo, the 180° refocusing pulse causes the water and fat MDM vectors to be in phase at a time interval from the 180° pulse equal to the time between the 180° pulse and the 90° pulse. Therefore, if we offset our signal measurement 2.25 mS either beyond or before this point in time, we will catch the water and fat MDM vectors exactly 180° out of phase, and their signals will cancel. Images produced in this fashion have the following property: each pixel representing a cancellation effect due to water-fat dephasing has a signal equal to water minus fat if the signal measurement is earlier than the re-focused echo; and fat minus water if the signal measurement is later. And if we do a standard spin-echo, then these same pixels will have a signal equal to water *plus* fat. Hence if we do an early offset, for example, we can get two equations in two unknowns for each of these pixels:

$$w + f = p_a$$
$$w - f = p_b$$

where w is the water signal, f is the fat signal, pb is the water minus fat signal measured in a pixel where there is dephasing, and pa is the water plus fat signal measured in this same pixel during the standard spin-echo sequence. Our two unknowns are w and f. And we can solve for w (the water signal) by adding the two equations; or we can solve for f (the fat signal) by subtracting the two equations. Hence we can obtain an image which effectively displays water and suppresses fat, and vice-versa. This is the method of Dixon.

It is important to realize that in the method of Dixon, fat and water interactions occur only in those pixels where fat and water molecules are contiguous to each other. This is different from the two other methods to be described later.

Now don't think that you can run to your scanner, do a spin-echo with a TE of 20 mS and then one with TE of 22.25 mS and then be able to do fat and water suppression. Even if you could set up the necessary math to solve for fat and water, it won't work. This is because in order to do the dephasing sequence, you must shift your read-out gradient (frequency) **relative** to the 180° pulse; and if you set up a sequence where TE = 22.25 mS on a standard scanner, you will shift **both** the 180° pulse and the read-out gradient, so that you will simply create another spin-echo sequence where water and fat are added. In other words, your scanner must be modified to offset signal measurement relative to the 180° refocusing pulse in order to obtain a water-minus-fat image for a spin-echo pulse sequence.

However, you *can* accomplish something like the method of Dixon with a gradient echo, or fast scan. Remember that in a fast scan, there is no 180° refocusing pulse. Hence all spins are in phase immediately after being flipped by the RF pulse; and they continue to dephase up to the time of signal measurement.* Hence fat and water MDM vectors are in phase every 4.5 mS and out of phase every other 2.25 mS (approximately). Therefore, a TE which is a multiple of 4.5 mS will essentially produce an in-phase water-plus-fat image, and a TE which is a multiple of 4.5 mS +2.25 mS will tend to produce a dephased water-minus-fat image. (There is no fat minus water image here). You may have actually seen a water-minus-fat fast scan image on an abdomen scan if you just happened to set up the right TE. In such an image, you would obtain a dark line surrounding each kidney representing dephasing of the water spins of the kidney with the neighboring fat spins of the perinephric fat. Of incidental interest, one vendor had referred to this phenomenon as chemical shift artifact "of the second kind". However, what we have described in this section is not a form of chemical shift artifact, but rather cancellation of signal due to dephasing.

Selective Spectral Excitation

In selective spectral excitation, we pre-saturate either water or fat MDM's in the following way: the usual spin-echo pulse cycle is prefaced by an additional 90° RF pulse that consists of a pure frequency equal to either that of water or fat. Remember that the only MDM's that are flipped by the RF pulse are those whose frequencies match the frequency of the RF pulse. Hence, to suppress fat, for example, we selectively flip the fat vectors 90° by using an RF frequency *exactly* equal to 64,000,220 Hz. (Once again, we are assuming that water precesses exactly at 64 MHz in a 1.5T magnet.) Then when the 2nd 90° pulse is applied, the fat vectors will be flipped a total of 180° and will yield no signal (fig. 19.5).

---

* Note that this is in spite of the gradient refocusing that we described in the section on fast scanning. That process is very different from the 180° refocusing pulse of a spin-echo sequence.

TIME ──────────────────────────►

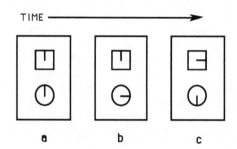

a   b   c

FIG. 19.5- SELECTIVE SPECTRAL EXCITATION
The square is a water MDM and the circle is a fat MDM. Point **a** is prior to the pulse cycle (both vectors at 12:00). At point **b**, a fat selective 90° RF pulse has been applied (water vector remains at 12:00; fat vector now at 3:00). At point **c**, the 2nd 90° RF pulse (non-selective) has been applied, and both vectors are shifted 90° (water vector now at 3:00; fat vector now at 6:00). Now the water vector has a signal because it is flipped a total of 90°, but the fat vector does not because it is flipped a total of 180°.

In practice, the fat selecting pulse is applied without a magnetic field gradient. The "regular" 90° RF pulse, which follows the fat selective pulse, consists of a mixture of fat and water frequencies, and is applied during the slice select gradient in the usual manner.

Note the striking similarity between this process and pre-saturation, which we described in the chapter on motion: for pre-saturation, we selectively saturated vectors outside the image volume, and in selective spectral excitation, we selectively saturate either water or fat vectors within the image volume.

Now there is a fundamental difference between fat suppressed images in the method of Dixon vs. fat suppressed images in selective spectral excitation. In the method of Dixon, the water-minus-fat images show regions of signal void where there are fat and water molecules adjacent to each other; whereas in selective spectral excitation, if fat is suppressed, for example, there will be a relative signal void wherever there is fat- even if there are no water molecules nearby.

Note that the method of Dixon and selective spectral excitation are often referred to as examples of "chemical shift imaging".

Summary of selective spectral excitation pulse cycle:

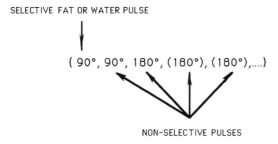

STIR Sequences

"STIR" is an acronym which stands for "Short **TI** **I**nversion **R**ecovery". It is an inversion recovery pulse sequence with a short inversion time (TI). Remember from our discussion of the inversion recovery pulse cycle in chapter 14 that after the magnetic vector M is flipped 180°, there is variable re-polarization of Mz depending on the T1 relaxation properties of the tissue. Remember also that fat has a shorter T1 than water. Therefore, if we use a relatively short inversion time, we will catch the fat Mz right at the 0 mark, whereas the Mz for water will still be partly inverted (fig. 19.6).

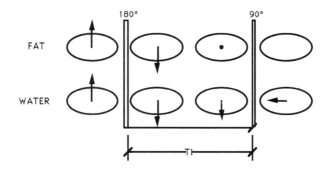

FIG. 19.6- STIR

Note that re-polarization of the fat Mz is more rapid than that for water. When the 90° "inversion" pulse is applied, the fat vector is 0, but the water vector still has a negative magnitude. Hence there is a resultant Mx signal in the x-y plane for water, but not for fat. Note that TI (time to invert) is the time interval between the 180° and 90° RF pulses, and is of the order of 100-200 mS, which is relatively short.

Then when the 90° pulse is applied, the inverted water Mz will be flipped into the x-y plane yielding a signal, whereas there is no fat Mz vector to flip, and hence there is no resulting Mx for fat. This effectively suppresses fat relative to water.

There are two things of note here. First, like the method of selective spectral excitation, fat tissue is suppressed wherever it is–not just where there is neighboring water tissue. Second, this is not one of the forms of chemical shift imaging, because the suppression principle here depends on differences in the T1 relaxation times of fat and water rather than differences in their MDM precession frequencies.

20
Coils

It may seem strange to discuss such a fundamental component of the MR scanner at the end of this book, but the author feels that even though it is important, it is peripheral to the structure of the fundamentals that we have covered up to this point.

There are three basic varieties of MR coils: (1) receiver, transmitter coils; (2) gradient coils; and (3) shim coils.

Receiver, Transmitter Coils

These are the most familiar of the MR coils. They do one or both of the following two things: (1) send or "broadcast" the RF pulse; and (2) receive or "pick up" the MR signal. In their simplest form, they are circular segments of wire with the ends of the wire attached to whatever is processing the signal or generating the pulse (fig. 20.1).

FIG. 20.1- SIMPLE COIL

There are usually three types of receiver and/or transmitter coils associated with an MR scanner: (1) the body coil; (2) the head coil; and (3) a variety of surface coils.

The body coil is a permanent part of the scanner, and surrounds the patient in much the same way as the helical coils of the magnet (neither of which is visible to the patient). The body coil is both a transmitter and receiver coil. The body coil's main function is to transmit the RF pulse for **all** scans, and to receive the MR signal only when imaging large parts of the body, such as the chest or abdomen.

The head coil is a semi-permanent component of the scanner and may or may not be detachable. It is usually an integral part of the helmet-like unit that the patient's head fits into when performing an MR scan of the brain. The head coil can be receiver only or both transmit and receiver.

Surface coils are separate devices that are attached to the scanner when needed by means of cables. There are a number of different surface coils corresponding to different parts of the body to be imaged: lumbar spine coils, knee coils, orbit coils, etc. Each has its own geometric design so that it may be applied as close to the body part to be imaged as possible. They are usually receiver-only coils, with the RF pulse again being supplied by the body coil; although a number of manufacturers are producing coils that transmit and receive.

The important concept regarding receiver or transmitter coils is that they are very much like TV or radio antennae. This means that where they are placed has nothing to do with the **spatial** characteristics of the image, only the strength of the signal. For example, if we mal-position a surface coil, the part being imaged will still appear in the proper place. However, its signal strength will be lessened, and there will be a poor signal-to-noise ratio. In general, a coil should be positioned as close to the part being examined as possible.

Gradient Coils

There are three sets of gradient coils, each oriented along one of the orthogonal axes. Their sole purpose is to produce an additional electromagnetic field which distorts the main external magnetic field thereby creating the gradients, which have already been discussed extensively. Incidentally, the pounding sound that one hears during an MR acquisition is caused by the gradient coils banging against the device that anchors them. In fact, one can count the number of slices by listening carefully to the pattern of the sounds!

Shim Coils

These coils are simply used to fine tune the main magnetic field so that it is homogeneous throughout the imaging volume.

Note that some of the state-of-the-art MRI scanners employ so-called "digital" coils. However, we will not discuss that topic here.

21
User Parameter Summary

It seems appropriate that the concluding chapter summarize all of the common parameters available to the user in terms of the various discussions in this book.

Anti-aliasing–used to prevent wrap-around in the phase encoding direction. When chosen, the exam time is lengthened.

Field of View–the area of tissue that is imaged. Can vary from less than 10 cm to about 60 cm. Smaller fields of view yield greater spatial resolution, but appear more grainy. Steeper gradients are used for smaller fields of view.

Frequency and Phase Encoding Directions–terminology varies with different vendors. Once the slice select axis is chosen, the user can determine which axis of the image plane is phase and which is frequency. This prerogative may be useful in eliminating wrap-around in the phase encoding direction.

Matrix Size–equal to the number of phase encoding steps (except for half-Fourier imaging); usually varies from 128 to 256. Larger matrices yield greater spatial resolution, but appear more grainy.

Number of Signal Averages–the number of pulse cycles per phase encoding step; usually varying from 1-8. More signal averages yield a less grainy image but take longer to acquire.

Projection–the user selects axial, coronal or sagittal, and this determines the slice select axis, which must be perpendicular to the selected plane.

RF Flip Angle–the number of degrees that the M vector is flipped from the vertical; usually 90° for spin echo sequences and less than 60° for fast scans. As the flip angle varies from 0° to 90°, the images become more T1 weighted and more signal rich

Slice Thickness–the thickness of the image slice; usually varies from 3-10 mm in 2DFT acquisitions, but may be thinner in 3DFT acquisitions. Thinner slices use steeper gradients and will appear more grainy.

TE–the time interval from flipping the M vector to measuring the signal; usually varies from 10-160 mS. Long TE's produce more T2 weighting (for spin-echo sequences), and short TE's produce more T1 weighting.

TR–the time interval between successive pulse cycles; usually varies from 20-3000 mS. Long TR's produce more T2 weighting (for spin-echo sequences), and short TR's produce more T1 weighting.

Bibliography

1. Anderson CM, Edelman RR, Turski PA, *Clinical Magnetic Resonance Angiography.* New York: Raven Press, 1993.

2. Balaban RS, Ceckler TL. Magnetization Transfer Contrast in Magnetic Resonance Imaging. *Magnetic Resonance Quarterly.* 1992; 8: 116-136.

3. Boas ML, *Mathematical Methods in the Physical Sciences.* New York: Wiley & Sons, 1966.

4. Bottomley PA, Foster TH, Argersinger RE, Pfeifer LM. A review of normal tissue hydrogen NMR relaxation times and relaxation mechanisms from 1-100 MHz: Dependence on tissue type, NMR frequency, temperature, species, excision, and age. *Am. Assoc. Phys. Med.* 1984; 425-448.

5. Bracewell RN, *The Fourier Transform and Its Applications.* 2nd ed. New York: McGraw-Hill, 1978.

6. Bradley WB. Flow Phenomena in MR Imaging. *AJR* 1988; 150: 983-993.

7. Curry TS, Dowdey JE, Murry RC. *Christensen's Introduction to the Physics of Diagnostic Radiology.* 3rd ed. Philadelphia: Lea & Febiger, 1984.

8. Edelman RR, Mattle HP, Atkinson DJ, Hoogewoud HM. MR Angiography. *AJR* 1990; 154: 937-946.

9. Feinberg DA, Hale JD, Watts JC, Kaufman L, Mark A. Halving MR Imaging Time by Conjugation. *Radiology* 1986; 161: 527-532.

10. Gomori JG, Holland GH, Grossman RI, Gefter WB, Lenkinski RE. Fat Suppression by Section-Select Gradient Reversal on Spin-Echo MR Imaging. *Radiology* 1988; 168: 493-495.

11. Granville WA, Smith PF, Longley WR, *Elements of the Differential and Integral Calculus.* Rev. ed. Boston: Ginn and Co., 1958.

12. Harms SE, Morgan TJ, Yamanashi WS, Harle TS, Dodd GD. Principles of nuclear magnetic resonance imaging. *Radiographics* 1984; 4: 26-43.

13. Richards JA, Sears FW, Wehr MR, Zemansky MW, *Modern University Physics*. Reading: Addison-Wesley, 1960.

14. Saini S, Frankel RB, Stark DD, Ferrucci JT, Magnetism: A primer and review. *AJR* 1988; 150: 735-744.

15. Stark DD, Bradley WG. *Magnetic Resonance Imaging*. St. Louis: C.V. Mosby, 1988.

16. Wehrli FW. Fast-Scan Magnetic Resonance. *Magnetic Resonance Quarterly* 1990; 6: 165-236.

17. Wood ML, Henkelman RM. MR image artifacts from periodic motion. *Med. Phys.* 1985; 12(2): 143-151.

Index